BRITISH SMALL ANIMAL VETERINARY ASSOCIATION

AN INTRODUCTION TO VETERINARY ANATOMY AND PHYSIOLOGY

by A. R. Michell B.Sc., B.Vet Med., Ph.D., M.R.C.V.S.
Dept. of Veterinary Medicine, Royal Veterinary College, University of London
and P. E. Watkins M.A., Vet M.B., Ph.D., D.V.R., M.R.C.V.S.
University of Bristol, Dept. of Anatomy, Park Row, Bristol, Avon BS1 5LS

Published by:

British Small Animal Veterinary Association
Kingsley House
Church Lane
Shurdington
Cheltenham
Gloucestershire
GL51 5TQ

First Published 1989
Reprinted 1993, 1997, 1998, 1999

Printed by:

Fusion Design
Fordingbridge
Hampshire

ISBN 0 905214 12 9

INTRODUCTION

This book aims to provide a simple first contact with veterinary anatomy and physiology. It does not set out to replace other textbooks or to be comprehensive. In particular, it is not concerned with research controversy, scientific evidence or even with access to background literature. In that sense it is self-contained – it is intended to be used and enjoyed in itself rather than directly followed up. However it recognises that students will need other books for examination purposes, and aims to make the reading of those books easier and more approachable.

The content of the book conforms to no specific examination syllabus. Nevertheless – or perhaps because of that – the book concentrates on matters which should be interesting and important to these involved in veterinary practice, whether as students, nurses or veterinary surgeons. It grew out of courses designed for the training of veterinary nurses but because it is deliberately direct rather than academic or comprehensive, we believe it will also be useful to a much wider audience. For this reason, we have called it simply "An Introduction to Veterinary Anatomy and Physiology". Since it is intended to help and interest its readers rather than demonstrate our scholarship we would greatly welcome comments on its clarity, content and usefulness.

A. R. Michell
P. E. Watkins

ACKNOWLEDGEMENTS

We would like to thank Rosemary Forster for preparing both the final manuscript and the index of this book and Ray Butcher for producing some of the illustrations. We would also like to thank Liz Watkins for her comments, criticism and advice.

AN INTRODUCTION TO VETERINARY ANATOMY AND PHYSIOLOGY
A. R. Michell and P. E. Watkins

Published by B.S.A.V.A.

Introduction

CHAPTER 1:
BASIC CONCEPTS

ANATOMY AND PHYSIOLOGY

Anatomy is concerned with the structure of the body – not only the visible structure but the underlying arrangement of the cells and even the minute organelles within them. Fundamentally, anatomy concerns the relationship between structure and function, for example between the shapes of bones, the muscles pulling on them and the way the animal moves – or the relationship between the shape of the molecules making up muscle protein, its visible structure under a microscope and the way it contracts.

Physiology is concerned with the functions of the body and, above all, with the way they are controlled. Like anatomy, it would ideally aim to explain all body functions in relation to the chemicals making up the molecular structure of cells and tissues. At that point it turns imperceptibly into biochemistry. Since both anatomy and physiology aim to explain the features of animals in relation to their molecular structure, they are, in a sense, different ways of looking at the same thing. Any animal looks and acts the way it does because its genes have enabled it to produce a particular range of proteins. Some of these contribute to its structure. Others, especially the enzymes, dominate the pattern of chemical reactions underlying the production of the structural components of the body and the processes which allow them to function.

This book is not just concerned with anatomy and physiology for their own sake but with the extent to which they enable us to understand, diagnose, prevent or treat clinical conditions. It is more concerned with visible anatomy as it relates to surgery or to physiological function and with how the major organs work, rather than with biochemical detail. Nor is it concerned with function within individual cells e.g. cell division or details of their components, e.g. nucleus, mitochondria, lysosomes, endoplasmic reticulum. Nevertheless neither anatomy nor physiology can really be understood without at least some outline biochemistry and cell physiology here and there.

7

ANATOMY: METHODS OF DESCRIPTION

When exploring the structure of the animal body we must be able to accurately describe the position of its many component parts. It is for this reason that we must learn certain anatomical terms which, although appearing rather cumbersome, will be very useful in the ensuing chapters.

The terms used are listed below, and are illustrated in Figures 1-1 and 1-2.

When considering the trunk of the body, the anatomical terms used are:

CRANIAL: meaning closer to the head, and
CAUDAL: meaning closer to the tail.

At the head the term ROSTRAL is used, which means closer to the muzzle.

DORSAL: meaning closer to the back of the trunk, and
VENTRAL: meaning closer to the belly.

MEDIAL: implying closer to the midline of the body, and
LATERAL: implying closer to the side of the body.
(Medial and Lateral are also used when describing the position of structures in the limbs).

In the limbs, additional anatomical terms are used:

PROXIMAL: meaning closer to the junction of the limb and the trunk, whereas structures situated at a distance in the limb are described as DISTAL. For example, in the forelimb, the elbow is more proximal than the toe.

Proximal to the carpus in the forelimb, and the hock in the hindlimb, the term CRANIAL indicates structures lying nearer the "front", and CAUDAL implies structures nearer the "rear".

Distal to the carpus the term DORSAL is used to indicate structures lying nearer the "front", those nearer the "rear" are PALMAR.

Distal to the hock, the term PLANTAR implies that a structure is closer to the "rear", and DORSAL again means closer to the "front".

It may be useful to refer back to this section, and the accompanying diagrams, at regular intervals as you study the rest of the book. This will help you to gain an understanding of the anatomical relationships of the various systems of the body, and of the components of each system. This will ensure that you understand the structure of the animal body and its importance in both health and disease.

PHYSIOLOGY: REGULATION

Physiology is basically about how the body works and the discoveries which support our explanations. Although these questions of scientific evidence are

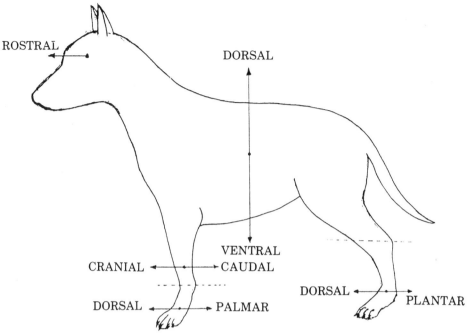

Figure 1-1. Lateral view of a dog to demonstrate anatomical directions.

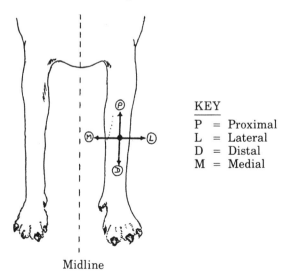

KEY

P = Proximal
L = Lateral
D = Distal
M = Medial

Figure 1-2. Cross-section of a dog at the level of the forelimb to demonstrate anatomical directions.

very important to pure physiologists, they will not concern us at all; this book seeks purely to explain, not to prove.

The keystone of physiology is regulation. Just as an aircraft needs to have its temperature, pressure, speed, and angle regulated to provide a safe and stable environment for its passengers the body regulates the concentration of its chemicals, the pressure of its blood, the temperature, the speed of breathing and many other functions. It thus provides a *stable internal environment* in which its cells can live and function efficiently.

For a clinician, whether a nurse or a vet, the issue goes beyond regulation itself, however, because we want, above all, to understand how regulation can become involved in disease, either by going wrong and causing it or by adapting and defending against its effects.

REGULATORY SYSTEMS: 'FEEDBACK'

Regulation does not just imply the ability to maintain constancy, though that is important. It also implies the ability to set the level of constancy, the target, appropriately for the animal's needs. A puppy and a dog each have a reasonably constant volume of fluid in their body day to day, but as the puppy grows the volume inevitably changes. A bitch needs a different body fluid volume during pregnancy or lactation. Body temperature changes during the reproductive cycle or even during the day but it is always regulated, i.e. there are mechanisms which at any given moment will correct any tendency to depart from a fixed target temperature or 'set point'. This corresponds to the thermostat setting in a heating system. If room temperature differs from set point action is automatically taken; the heating is switched on or off as appropriate. This simple control system needs

    (a) Receptors   – to measure whatever is regulated

    (b) Effectors   – to alter whatever is regulated

and (c) A set point   – or target value of whatever is regulated.

There also needs to be 'feedback' of information from the receptors to allow the current value of what is being regulated to be compared with 'set point' and appropriate action triggered if they differ. The response *reduces the change which triggered it*, e.g. a rise in temperature, above set point, triggers cooling. Such a system maintains stability and is called a *negative feedback* system (the response is negative to the disturbance). Most physiological regulation involves negative feedback.

Occasionally we encounter systems in which responses *amplify or perpetuate the disturbance* – like power steering in a car. Such a system is obviously not stable but it is useful e.g. to accelerate the emptying of the bladder during micturition or the uterus during parturition. These are examples of *positive feedback*. Such systems are less common in physiology but they frequently develop as features of disease – another description of a positive feedback system could be a vicious circle. Nothing better illustrates the replacement of stable negative feedback regulation by vicious circles or positive feedback than the development of circulatory shock (Chapter 6).

The sum total of the processes keeping the various regulated aspects of body function constant is called 'homeostasis', the maintenance of a stable internal environment. Although the words 'regulate' and 'control' are interchangeable in everyday English, they have a slight difference of meaning in physiology. Any process which can be changed from one level to another can be controlled. Pressing the accelerator, brakes or turning the steering wheel all control various features of a car's performance, ultimately its speed and direction. But all could equally be controlled by a blindfolded driver. The driver's role is to add regulation to control: to use the controls to achieve the target direction and speed of the car and to correct deviations from set point. We can only do this if we have feedback – if we can see – to compare present speed and direction with set point.

Thus the body can clearly control its blood pressure (Chapter 6) or temperature (Chapter 4) – it merely needs the sympathetic nerves to alter the setting of the blood vessels or hormones to increase heat production. What converts this into regulation is the body's ability to measure the outcome, i.e. to detect pressure and temperature and, more important, to compare them with the current target of constancy, i.e. the 'set point'. Most physiological systems respond to several types of change or have several ways of responding. But then, even a heating system may well respond to temperature changes in several places, and control several functions e.g. heating, air conditioning and ventilation. Indeed the additional sophistication of measurement and response is likely to make it more effective in achieving satisfactory regulation.

UNDERSTANDING PHYSIOLOGY

Physiology is, above all, about systems, i.e. about components of the body which interact in a predictable and intelligible fashion. About the increase in heart rate which follows a haemorrhage, for example; we can understand both why it occurs and why it 'makes sense'. It is entirely possible to 'learn' the pages of a physiology textbook perfectly, like school poetry, yet understand nothing. The aim of learning physiology is to understand the system sufficiently to explain or predict its responses to common or important disturbances – whether caused by everyday life, disease, or its treatment. When it is really understood we can say 'I could construct a diagram or a model to explain how that works' – not copy, or remember but construct, because I understand. That is not to say that learning is unimportant – you cannot understand something unless you know a certain amount about it. But detail is never the objective in itself; the objective is to truly understand. When you do understand, you should be able to explain it to an intelligent school leaver, in your own words.

CHAPTER 2:
THE SKIN

An understanding of the structure and function of normal skin is necessary for all those involved in veterinary medicine. Skin diseases form a considerable proportion of the caseload seen in general veterinary practice. In addition, to gain access to the body (either for an intravenous injection, or for a surgical operation) one must cross the skin.

FUNCTIONS

The functions of the skin are:

1. Protection

The skin is the dividing layer between the "controlled" internal environment of the body, and the potentially "hostile" external environment. It prevents the loss of water and electrolytes from the internal environment and prevents absorption of toxic and harmful substances from the external environment. The intact skin prevents entrance of pathogens (harmful micro-organisms) into the body; it also protects the body from mechanical trauma. Part of the protection against pathogens results from the presence on skin of a normal "flora" of harmless bacteria which compete with abnormal and potentially harmful bacteria and thus restrain their growth. The normal flora of the gut gives protection in a similar fashion. Obviously skin is seldom sterile, i.e. free from micro-organisms – hence the importance of cleansing before injection or surgery.

2. Production

Vitamin D is required for the absorption of calcium from the intestine. It is synthesised in the skin by the action of ultra-violet light on a precursor chemical. The vitamin D produced is not metabolically active until it has undergone further chemical changes in the liver and kidneys.

Secretions produced by different glands in the skin pass out to the skin surface; these include:

13

(a) Sebum, produced by sebaceous glands, is an oily secretion which forms a thin, water-repellent layer over the skin; it imparts a sheen to the coat and helps control bacterial growth on the skin surface.

(b) Sweat, a watery secretion produced by sweat glands which is important in some animals as a means for thermoregulation.

(c) Milk, produced by mammary glands, is a source of nutrients for the newborn animal.

(d) Pheromones, produced by specialised skin glands, play a role in communication between animals (Chapter 11).

3. Sensory

The body must be able to monitor the external environment which surrounds it. This is achieved, in part, by sensory nerve receptors located in the lower part of the skin (the dermis). The receptors may respond to four basic stimuli:

Touch
Pain
Temperature
Pressure

Leading from the receptors are nerve fibres which pass to the spinal cord.

4. Storage

Fat is stored in the lower layers of the skin as adipose tissue, also called subcutaneous fat. This is both an energy store and a thermal insulating layer (Chapter 4). The amount of subcutaneous fat varies between animals; this can be seen by comparing a racing Greyhound with a "portly" Labrador.

In general, the factors which influence the amount of subcutaneous fat are:
(a) Age: Young animals have very small amounts of subcutaneous fat.

(b) Diet: When food is in ample supply, the body stores fat as an "insurance policy" against possible future shortages.

(c) Physical fitness: Athletic animals have very small amounts of subcutaneous fat.

(d) Environmental temperature: Animals living in cold environments deposit fat which provides thermal insulation.

The presence of excessive subcutaneous fat is often a hindrance, both to the palpation of structures lying below the skin (e.g. the superficial arteries for assessment of the peripheral pulse) and to the exposure of the body's internal organs at the time of surgery.

5. Thermoregulation

The skin plays an important role in thermoregulation, primarily by preventing heat loss from the body.

Blood flow to the skin can be reduced by vasoconstriction (contraction of smooth muscle in the walls of blood vessels). This reduces the amount of heat energy which is lost from the skin.

Erection of hair traps a layer of still air next to the skin, this provides a further layer of thermal insulation, similar to the effect of double-glazing of windows.

Subcutaneous fat acts as an insulating layer.

Heat may also be lost from the skin by sweating. However this is a relatively unimportant method of thermoregulation in the dog and cat (Chapter 4).

6. Communication

Pheromones are natural scents, produced e.g. by specialised skin glands and used for communication between animals of the same species. An example is the secretions produced by the anal glands and stored in the anal sacs; these are passed out of the body at the time of defaecation, and appear to play a role in the marking of territory.

An example of visual communication involving the skin is seen if an animal is threatened (be it by another animal or a person). It will respond by erecting the hairs of its coat (raising its "hackles"), so appearing much larger than it actually is!

STRUCTURE

The skin forms a covering layer over the body, being continuous with the mucous membranes of the nares, mouth, anus and genital openings. It is

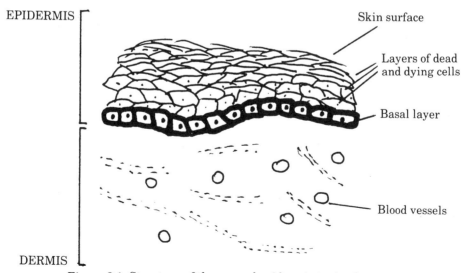

Figure 2-1. Structure of the normal epidermis in the dog.

15

composed of two layers, the outer epidermis and the underlying dermis, which is supported on a layer of connective tissue, called the subcutis, or hypodermis.

EPIDERMIS

This is composed of dead and dying cells arranged in a series of layers. Cells are produced at the basal layer (Fig. 2-1), and migrate up to the skin surface. During this migration the cells die, and a protein, keratin, is deposited in them. Dead cells are continually being lost to the external environment from the skin surface and constitute the scurf normally seen on an animal's coat. The epidermis is usually thickest in areas subjected to the greatest mechanical wear and tear; for example, the footpads. Long-term mechanical trauma to the skin will cause thickening of the epidermis. This explains the development of calluses, often seen on the lateral aspect of the elbows of large dogs which lie on rough surfaces.

There are no blood vessels in the epidermis, and the cells of the basal layer receive their nutrients by diffusion from the underlying dermis.

DERMIS

The dermis is composed of fibrous connective tissue which contains a variety of blood vessels, nerves and sensory receptors, muscles, hair follicles, glands and pigment cells.

The connective tissue of the dermis provides further mechanical protection, and it is usually thickened in areas subjected to greatest mechanical forces, e.g. footpads. Elastic tissue is also present in the dermis and acts as a "shock absorber". An important property of skin is the ability to repair wounds. The initial protection comes from the scab formed by blood clotting (Chapter 5) but then, beneath this, the true repair occurs, involving both dermis and epidermis.

HAIR

A characteristic of the mammals is a covering of hair over the skin. Most dogs and cats have a thick coat covering nearly all the skin surface. There are, however, a few regions where the hair cover is very thin, examples are at the nipples of the mammary glands, and the skin around the anus. Hair is composed of keratin, plus pigments. It grows from the base of a small tube, called a hair follicle (Fig. 2-2). The hair follicle originates from the epidermis and grows down into the underlying dermis. Attached to the deeper section of the hair follicle is a small band of smooth muscle called the arrector pili muscle.

Contraction of this muscle causes the hair to become erect (piloerection).

Closely associated with the hair follicle, and opening into it, is a sebaceous gland. The sebum produced by the gland is released into the hair follicle and then passes out onto the skin surface.

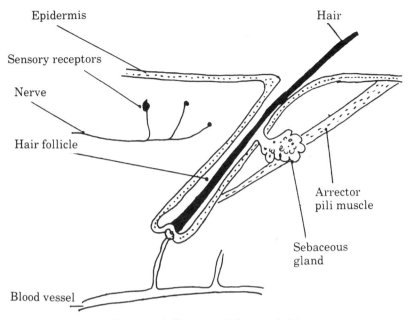

Figure 2-2. Structure of normal skin.

Hair growth follows a cyclical pattern, with periods of active growth followed by periods of hair loss. A number of factors, both internal (e.g. nutritional) and environmental, influence hair growth. Hormones affect the hair cycle, and this explains why some hormonal disorders may lead to abormalities of hair growth. For example, in hypothyroidism there are reduced levels of thyroxine which leads to hair loss, primarily from around the flanks and thighs.

There are specialised long tactile hairs on the head. These are called vibrissae or whiskers, and are found in the skin of the upper and lower jaws, and above the eye. They detect mechanical stimuli.

SKIN GLANDS

There are numerous glands associated with the skin, which produce a variety of secretions.

Sebaceous glands produce sebum; its function has been discussed earlier. In certain skin diseases, there is production of an excessive amount of sebum, which leads to a greasy skin; this is the condition of seborrhoea.

The circumanal glands lie in the hairless skin around the anus, and open onto the overlying skin. Their secretion is believed to include a pheromone. In older male dogs the glands commonly undergo benign enlargement, leading to the condition of perianal adenomata. Enlargement of the glands in this condition is stimulated by the male hormone testosterone; this explains why castration (removal of the testes) is used in the treatment of this condition.

17

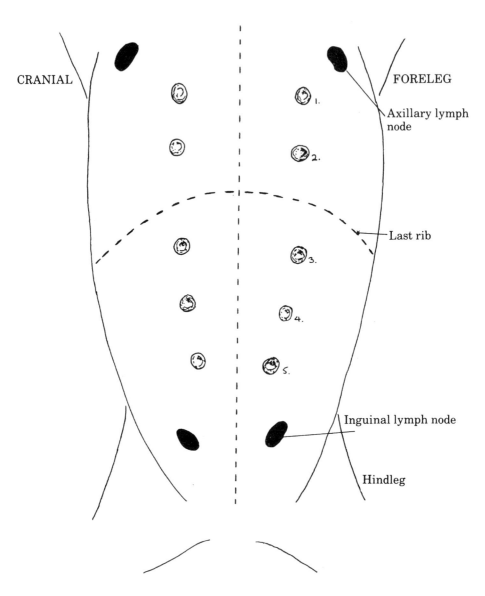

CRANIAL

FORELEG

Axillary lymph node

1.

2.

Last rib

3.

4.

5.

Inguinal lymph node

Hindleg

Key: 1: Cranial thoracic gland
2: Caudal thoracic gland
3: Cranial abdominal gland
4: Caudal abdominal gland
5: Inguinal gland
In the cat, the caudal abdominal glands are absent.

Figure 2-3. Distribution of mammary glands in the dog.

18

Although sweating is a relatively unimportant method of thermoregulation in the dog and cat, sweat glands are found at certain sites in the skin. The commonest is the footpads where sweat glands open directly onto the skin's surface.

Mammary glands are specialised skin glands, and are another characteristic of mammals. The mammary glands are positioned on the ventral body wall over the thorax and abdomen on either side of the midline (Fig. 2-3). The dog normally possesses five pairs of glands, the cat four pairs. Mammary glands are present in both the male and female, but normally only enlarge and produce milk in the female. Development of mammary glands is under hormonal control, with oestrogens playing an important role (Chapters 9 and 13). High levels of oestrogens in the male will cause mammary enlargement, often with milk production. Perhaps most disconcerting (especially for the owner) is that this may occur in certain cases of testicular tumours!

Each mammary gland normally has one teat (nipple), although occasionally there may be two. The teat has multiple openings (orifices) which lead into a branching network of ducts and sinuses finally terminating in the glandular tissue (Fig. 2-4). Milk produced by the gland is stored in the ducts and sinuses. In response to the hormone oxytocin (Chapter 9) there is contraction of smooth muscle in the wall of the ducts causing expulsion of milk.

Tumours of the mammary gland are not uncommon in the bitch and many are malignant. These may spread (metastasise) to the local lymph nodes (the axillary node cranially, and the superficial inguinal node caudally; Fig. 2-3). In addition, they may spread to the lungs. This explains the need to radiograph the thorax (to assess the presence or absence of secondary tumours) prior to attempting surgical removal of a mammary tumour.

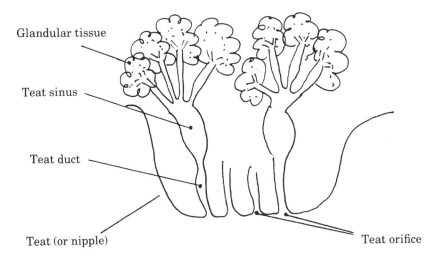

Figure 2-4. Structure of the mammary gland of the dog.

Milk is the source of nutrients for the newborn and young animal. The first milk produced following parturition is called colostrum, and this contains immunoglobulins (Chapter 5) which are proteins involved in providing immunity. These are absorbed directly from the intestine into the bloodstream of the newborn animal. It is vital that all newborn animals receive an adequate amount of colostrum; failure to do so places the animal at risk of infection.

FOOTPADS

Footpads are the major load-bearing surfaces of the feet. Both the epidermis and dermis are markedly thickened in these areas. The footpad is hairless.

At the forepaw there is a large metacarpal pad which lies over the distal section of the metacarpus; and four digital footpads; one pad for each weight-bearing digit. There is also a carpal pad, sited over the caudal aspect of the carpal joint; this does not normally bear weight.

At the hindpaw, there is one metatarsal pad (situated over the distal part of the metatarsal region) plus four digital pads.

CLAWS

Claws are composed of modified epidermis and cover part of the distal phalanx (or toe bone). There is one claw per digit. They play a role in locomotion by weight-bearing; they are also used for fighting and for obtaining food. Claws are beak shaped, being flattened from side to side and in cats they can be retracted into a sheath. The wall of the claw is made of a hard, horny material. The dermis lies at the base of the claw; it is highly vascular and has structural connections with the outer layer (periosteum) of the distal phalanx. Over-zealous claw clipping will easily expose the dermis and can lead to bleeding. Normal weight-bearing leads to gradual wear of the claws, which continue to grow throughout life. Failure of normal wear leads to lengthening of the claw which, because of its curved shape, may grow into the digital footpad.

On the medial aspect of the metacarpal (and occasionally metatarsal) region there may be a small, non-weight-bearing digit; this is the dew-claw. This is a vestige of the first digit (the thumb in man) and is more commonly found in the foreleg than the hindleg. Since the digit is not weight-bearing the dew-claw is not worn down and may grow into the neighbouring skin. Dew-claws are commonly removed from puppies soon after birth to prevent this problem arising.

CHAPTER 3:
THE THORAX, BREATHING AND RESPIRATION

INTRODUCTION: WHAT IS RESPIRATION?

Unfortunately the scientific meaning of respiration is different from the ordinary everyday meaning. Strictly, the scientific meaning of respiration relates to the chemical processes allowing cells to obtain energy from raw materials (substrates) derived from food. Digestion (Chapter 8) is about the conversion of food into useful substances (for various purposes, not just respiration). Respiration is about the cellular use of substrates to obtain energy. The ordinary English meaning of respiration refers purely to one aspect of the process – the delivery of oxygen (which is usually needed for respiration) and the removal of waste CO_2 which is always an end product.

Cells can hoard energy for various uses just as we can bank money to use for various purposes. Equally, cells can obtain energy in several ways – just as there are various ways of making money. The energy obtained is not created (only nuclear physicists can actually create energy!) it is merely transferred from one chemical to another (just as we don't *literally* 'make' money – we exchange it). The significance of money is that it is a currency; it circulates between people and links a variety of services to a variety of purchases in an agreed, predictable way. Similarly, there is a 'currency' in energy metabolism which is the chemical called ATP (adenosine triphosphate). It can be made in various ways and used for almost any purpose requiring energy (movement, chemical reactions, heat production, etc.). The most common substrates obtained from digestion which can be used to produce ATP are glucose and fatty acids. They are not made into ATP but energy is transferred from chemical reactions involving them into reactions converting ADP (adenosine diphosphate) into ATP (just as the sale of a TV does not convert it into money but allows money to be stored). ATP is like a high bank balance; it can be spent to liberate energy. ADP is like a low bank balance; it needs to be topped up with energy (ADP converted back into ATP) to allow further expenditure.

There are two main ways of obtaining ATP in the body – which are really different branches of a single pathway. One is aerobic – needs oxygen in its final stages – and creates lots of energy (ATP). In the absence of oxygen an earlier branch in the chemical pathway becomes a diversion which still allows ATP to be produced, but only very inefficiently, in small amounts and at the sacrifice of generating lots of acid (lactic acid – what you smell in sour milk and one of the factors that makes your muscles feel stiff after a hard sprint). Really this is an 'emergency' or 'standby' way of operating – it can not go on for long and some cells can hardly manage it at all, without danger (brain). As soon as oxygen is restored the chemicals accumulating in the branch line (mainly acid) are diverted back into the main line allowing oxygen to be used to restore the depleted stores of ATP. That gets rid of the lactic acid (and it is why you breathe harder after a sprint than while you are running). You will learn a little more about those chemical pathways in Chapter 8 (on digestion), and in Chapter 12 you will learn that muscle has a secondary energy store (creatine phosphate) that it can use to bolster its ATP (like having some dollars to convert into pounds in an emergency).

The rest of this Chapter is about respiration in the ordinary everyday – and clinical – sense, i.e. the processes allowing efficient gas exchange in the lungs. Without this removal of CO_2 from the blood and constant replenishment of the circulating oxygen, cellular respiration would cease; starved of supplies and depressed by accumulated waste products. Of course, even if the lungs work perfectly cells will be in just as much trouble if the circulation of the blood is inefficient. The respiratory system (thoracic wall, diaphram, lungs and airways) prepares the blood for re-delivery to the tissues but that delivery depends on the circulatory system (Chapter 6).

PULMONARY EXCHANGE

Air is rich in oxygen (20%) and sparse in carbon dioxide (less than 0.01%). Nature does not allow unequal concentrations within spaces in good contact. Therefore carbon dioxide (CO_2) which is plentiful in blood diffuses (moves into less occupied space) into the air in the lungs. Oxygen (which is plentiful in the air) diffuses into the blood (which has become oxygen depleted by the activity of the body tissues). The expired air has 400 times as much CO_2 (4%) and, correspondingly, its oxygen has fallen by 4% (to 16%). This replenishment of blood oxygen and removal of carbon dioxide in the lungs is called pulmonary exchange.

In the tissues, oxygen is used up and CO_2 is produced, therefore oxygen is more plentiful in blood and again it diffuses towards the lower concentration of the tissue; the blood unloads its oxygen. Since the tissues are producing CO_2, that diffuses towards the lower concentration in blood. The blood becomes loaded with CO_2. The process is the exact opposite of what occurs in the lungs (Fig. 3-1).

It is just as important that oxygen is properly carried and unloaded otherwise there is no point in acquiring it efficiently in the lungs. Transport is achieved by the binding of oxygen to the haemoglobin of the red cells of the blood (RBC, erythrocytes). Much more 0_2 is carried than could freely dissolve in water. Fortunately, haemoglobin picks up oxygen best when blood CO_2 is falling (as in the lungs) and liberates it best when CO_2 and acidity are rising (i.e. in the tissues).

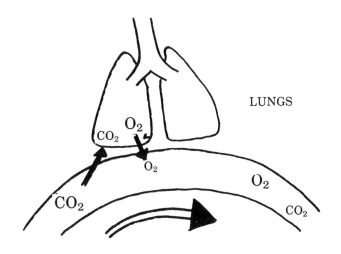

LUNGS

O_2

CO_2

O_2

O_2

CO_2

CO_2

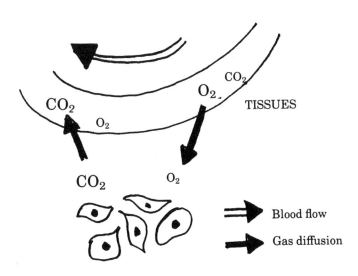

CO_2

O_2

TISSUES

CO_2

O_2

CO_2

O_2

Blood flow

Gas diffusion

Figure 3-1. Gas exchange in lungs and tissues

Anaemia is a lack of haemoglobin – not enough RBC, destruction of RBC, or not enough haemoglobin in each RBC. Even though there is less haemoglobin the animal can compensate by circulating it faster, i.e. by having a higher resting heart rate. It will not, therefore, be disadvantaged at rest or even in moderate activity. At high levels of activity the anaemic animal is disadvantaged because there is no escape from the fact that its maximum heart rate will deliver less oxygen while it has less haemoglobin to carry it.

When haemoglobin is heavily depleted of oxygen it becomes blue and this is observed in mucous membranes as cyanosis. Usually it does not become that depleted, even in the tissues, so although venous blood is a less bright red than arterial blood, it is certainly not blue. If circulation is very sluggish, cyanosis can occur because the tissues use oxygen at their normal rate but receive it more slowly. Anaemia does not cause cyanosis because less oxygen is delivered but there is less haemoglobin to become blue. Congenital defects of the heart or great vessels may allow some venous blood to bypass the lungs and enter the arterial circulation without reloading with oxygen. The tissues then receive blood containing haemoglobin that already has less oxygen than normal; by the time the tissues have extracted their oxygen, the haemoglobin is sufficiently unloaded (desaturated) to cause cyanosis – as in 'blue' babies!

You might wonder why the tissues do not obtain all the oxygen from haemoglobin – it seems a waste to leave so much behind in venous blood. But oxygen will only travel (diffuse) 'downhill' along a concentration gradient, i.e. for the blood oxygen to be reduced almost to nothing in the capillaries, the tissues would need an even lower oxygen. Only then could the last of the blood oxygen reach them from the capillaries (by diffusion). At such low oxygen levels the tissues would be dead!

The loading of haemoglobin in the lungs, on the other hand, is normally complete, over quite a range of oxygen concentrations in air. Additional breathing, therefore, cannot produce higher levels of oxygen in the blood – though it will provide for full oxygenation of a faster bloodflow through the lungs, after exercise for example.

Transport of carbon dioxide in blood is much easier. A little is simply dissolved, about a quarter binds to haemoglobin but most not only dissolves but reacts with water in the red cells to form carbonic acid (because RBC's have an enzyme, called carbonic anhydrase, which accelerates this reaction). Like any acid, this splits (dissociates) to yield hydrogen ions (H^+) and, in this case, bicarbonate (or hydrogen carbonate) ions, HCO_3^- (see also Chapter 7). Thus most carbon dioxide travels in the form of bicarbonate but is released as CO_2 in the lungs. Just as CO_2 helped the loading of oxygen in the lungs, oxygen encourages the unloading of CO_2. Equally, the unloading of oxygen from blood in tissue capillaries makes it easier for CO_2 to be loaded.

When animals are mainly metabolising (using) carbohydrate, they produce as much CO_2 as the oxygen they use. But when they mainly use fat, more of the oxygen ends up as water and less as CO_2, therefore oxygen is used faster than CO_2 is produced.

All that we have said about pulmonary exchange assumes, so far, that air is just there, ready to exchange gases with blood. The process of ensuring that

24

air arrives in the tiny thin-walled air sacs of the lungs (the alveoli) in sufficient quantities to replenish the blood, depends not only on breathing but on its proper regulation.

REGULATION OF BREATHING

Breathing is controlled (subconsciously) to achieve replacement of alveolar air sufficiently frequently to maintain a normal CO_2 concentration in blood. If blood CO_2 rises, we breathe harder and get rid of the excess. If blood CO_2 falls, we breathe slower and/or shallower to allow it to rise. Either way, blood CO_2 returns to its normal (set point) value. The receptors monitoring (detecting) the blood CO_2 are on the surface of a particular area of the brain. This is important because not only would a high CO_2 suggest poor oxygenation (i.e. inadequate exchange of both O_2 and CO_2) and a particular threat to brain cells, low CO_2 directly depresses brain blood flow. (This is why deliberate overbreathing can cause loss of consciousness.)

As an emergency back-up, there are also receptors in the main arterial supply to the brain (the carotids) which detect the oxygen concentration in blood and respond if it is inadequate. So although the adequacy of gas exchange (and breathing) is mainly ensured by a constant check on CO_2 levels, if, despite this, blood oxygen should fall, additional receptors trigger increased breathing. Although it is simple and adequate to think of blood O_2 and CO_2 in terms of concentration, you will encounter terms like 'tension' or 'partial pressure' of these gases. Essentially these just look at the same thing by saying what gas mixture would produce those concentrations. So if dry air was at 750 mm Hg pressure and had 20% oxygen, the partial pressure or tension of oxygen would be 750/5, i.e. 150 mm Hg. The oxygen tension of alveolar air is less than this, because oxygen is constantly being extracted into blood (and because air also contains water vapour) but the oxygen tension in arteria ood is almost identical to alveolar air.

The movement of air in and out of the lungs is called pulmonary ventilation and the amount of air moved depends on both the rate and depth of breathing. The rate and rhythm are set by the brain (subconsciously) in accordance with the CO_2 and O_2 receptors already described and signals from the lungs themselves (to prevent overstretching or to produce the protective exaggerated expiration of coughing).

PULMONARY VENTILATION

Functionally, the chest cavity (thorax) is a sealed cone entered by the trachea at its narrow end and walled off from the abdomen by the diaphragm at its wide end. During inspiration the volume of the chest cavity expands because of the change in shape of the rib cage (achieved by the intercostal muscles) and the flattening of the diaphragm from its normal dome shape. Obviously as the chest expands the pressure within it drops; air must therefore enter via the trachea and expand the lungs to keep pace with the expansion of the chest.

The object of this is to fill the microscopic sacs called alveoli which, with their thin moist walls, allow easy exchange of gases between air and blood. The air reaches them via the trachea, bronchi and bronchioles which, since they conduct air but do not allow gas exchange, are known as the dead space. (There is additional dead space in the upper respiratory tract.) Clearly each inspiration of air through the nostrils must fill the dead space before it can fill the alveoli. The deeper the breath, the more of it is available for the alveoli. If breathing were very shallow, each volume of inspired air would merely be enough to replenish the dead space, without reaching the alveoli at all. Pulmonary exchange (CO_2 and O_2 exchange) would then cease despite the work done in breathing. This leads to two important conclusions:

(a) A certain level of pulmonary ventilation could be achieved either by breathing shallow but fast or slow but deep; the latter would allow greater gas exchange. Dogs exploit this when they pant. They move more air to cool themselves (Chapter 4) but, by breathing faster and shallower, they do so with minimal disturbance to the actual gas exchange.

(b) If dead space is increased, less of the air taken in at each breath is available to the alveoli. Anaesthetic tubes are, in effect, external extensions of the trachea since the actual fresh air (or oxygen) begins where they reach the atmosphere or the rebreathing bag. The total length of tubing, therefore, needs to be as short as possible, especially in the very small animals.

Inspiration requires muscular work by the intercostals and diaphragm. Breathing out (expiration) is passive, i.e. requires no additional effort. The elastic energy stored in the expanded chest and, above all, in the expanded lungs, is sufficient to collapse them automatically, like a balloon. Only if disease has made the lungs less elastic or if the airway is obstructed does expiration require effort. Then the effort may be audible as a grunt. The entire process described hinges on the sole entry for air being via the trachea. If air can find an alternative way into the chest cavity, e.g. via a wound (as in 'pneumothorax') expansion of the chest will fail to expand the lungs properly, which may collapse.

Having considered how the respiratory system works, we need to look in a little more detail at the structures which allow it to function.

ANATOMY OF THE RESPIRATORY SYSTEM

The respiratory tract may conveniently be divided into two major components:

The Conducting System

The Exchange Sites.

THE CONDUCTING SYSTEM

Dogs and cats are predominantly nose breathers, with inspired gas passing through the external nares into the nasal cavity. This is situated in the head, dorsal to the oral cavity (mouth) (Fig. 3-2). It is protected by the overlying nasal, frontal and maxillary bones. Inside the nasal cavity there are a large number of fine bony scrolls, called turbinates, which are covered by a mucous membrane. The turbinates have a very good blood supply, so local trauma, or

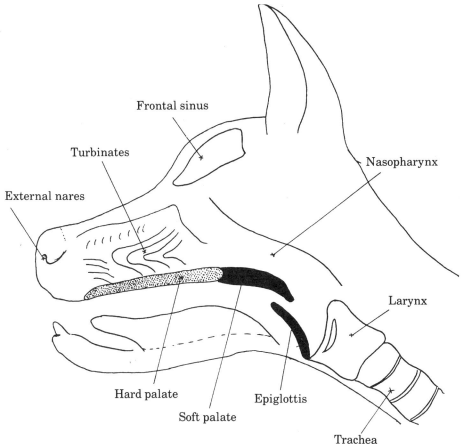

Figure 3-2. Longitudinal section of the nasal cavity and larynx.

infection, often leads to profuse haemorrhage. (This is manifest clinically as nose-bleeding, also called epistaxis.) As the inspired air passes over the turbinates it is humidified (moistened) and warmed; this reduces the loss of water and heat from the lungs. The complicated shape of the upper respiratory tract also helps to filter out particles, including bacteria, and so protects the lungs.

The mucous membrane of the nasal cavity contains a large number of nerve endings responsive to smell. This "special sense" (also called olfaction) is highly developed in both cats and dogs (Chapter 11). Irritation of the nasal mucous membrane, either by physical or chemical agents, causes sneezing, an important protective mechanism which prevents the animal from inhaling foreign or noxious material.

The clinical signs observed in animals with nasal disease include difficulty in breathing, sneezing, nasal discharge (often containing blood) and poor appetite due to a loss of sense of smell.

The frontal sinuses are air-filled bony outpouchings from the nasal cavity, extending caudo-dorsally into the frontal bone. Their precise function is unclear, but nasal disease can spread to involve these structures.

Inspired air passes caudally from the nasal cavity into the pharynx; this area is common to both the respiratory and digestive systems. The opening from the nasal cavity into the pharynx can be temporarily closed by contraction and elevation of the soft palate. This normally occurs when food is swallowed (Chapter 8), preventing food material from passing into the nasal cavity. Disruption of either the structure and/or function of the soft palate will prevent this occurring and can lead to food accumulating in the nasal cavity.

Air may also reach the pharynx via the mouth; this occurs when an animal is mouth-breathing. This allows a greater volume of air to be drawn into the

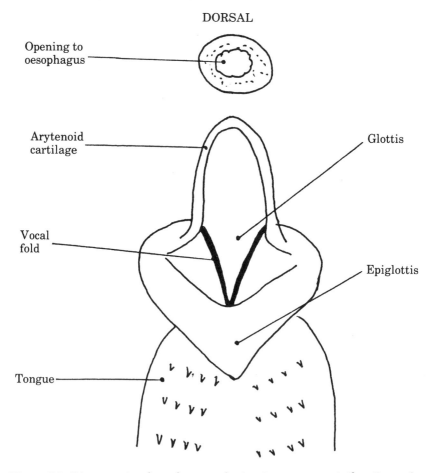

Figure 3-3. Diagram to show laryngeal structures seen at the time of endotracheal intubation.

lungs each minute. Mouth-breathing occurs when animals are performing strenuous exercise or when panting. It may occur at rest if there is an obstruction of the nasal cavity (e.g. by a tumour).

The larynx is the next component of the conducting system, and lies at the cranial end of the trachea. It is basically a box composed of numerous plates of cartilage joined together by small muscles and ligaments. The entrance into the larynx is called the glottis; its diameter can be varied (by means of muscular contraction) to help control airflow to the lungs.

It is very important that food in the pharynx does not enter the larynx so when an animal swallows, the glottis is closed. In addition, the epiglottis (the most rostral of the laryngeal cartilages) moves caudally to act as a lid to the glottis. Although the primary function of the larynx is to control airflow through the trachea, it also serves in the production of sound (phonation). The vocal folds form the lateral boundaries of the glottis and their vibration by air generates sound. The pitch of sound generated may be altered by adjusting the tension in the vocal folds.

The epithelium lining the larynx responds to irritation by rapid closure of the glottis (by means of a local reflex). This reflex is particularly well developed in the cat.

When introducing an endotracheal tube (to allow maintenance of general anaesthesia by gaseous agents) it is important to be familiar with the local anatomy. The tube is introduced via the mouth and passed into the pharynx. At this stage the soft palate must be displaced dorsally and the epiglottis displaced ventrally (using either a laryngoscope or the tube itself). This should allow the larynx to be seen, and most importantly the glottis can be observed; its diameter is seen to increase on inspiration. The end of the tube must be passed through the glottis, between the vocal folds, and into the trachea (Fig. 3-3). The tube can only be introduced correctly when the glottis is open. As a note of caution, it is easy for the endotracheal tube to be positioned incorrectly and to lie within the oesophagus which is situated dorsal to the larynx.

From the larynx the trachea runs caudally in the neck, passes between the first ribs and into the chest. At the level of the fifth rib the trachea divides into the primary bronchi (singular: bronchus) which pass into the lungs (Fig. 3-4). Of the two lungs, the right is larger than the left. Each lung is composed of a number of lobes (four in the right lung, three in the left).

The lumen (cavity) of the trachea is kept open by a series of incomplete U-shaped cartilage rings within its wall. The lining of the trachea contains a large number of cilia; these are small (microscopic) hairs which help trap foreign particles and transport them back up to the larynx where they are coughed out. (The cilia function in a similar way to an escalator). Irritation of the tracheal lining causes coughing. In the tracheal wall there are collections of lymphoid cells; these are part of the immune system and produce antibodies (Chapter 5) which are secreted into the lumen of the trachea and provide immunity against infection (e.g. kennel cough).

Structural support for a bronchus is provided by complete rings of cartilage in its wall. Each primary bronchus divides into a number of secondary bronchi

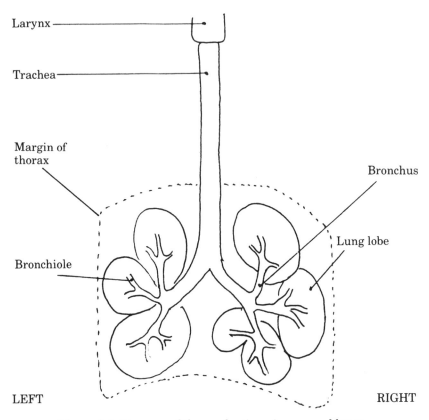

Larynx

Trachea

Margin of
thorax

Bronchiole

LEFT

Bronchus

Lung lobe

RIGHT

Figure 3-4. Diagram of the conducting airways and lungs.

within the lung. Further divisions of the secondary bronchi give rise to the small respiratory bronchioles and from these arise alveolar ducts leading down to the alveoli.

It is worth repeating that the components of the conducting system DO NOT play a role in gaseous exchange, and the volume of gas present in the conducting system is called the dead space. Connecting an animal to an anaesthetic circuit effectively increases the dead space and may significantly reduce the efficiency of breathing.

THE EXCHANGE SITES

Gaseous exchange takes place only at the alveoli. Each alveolus is a small sac which has a very thin epithelium. As a result, air in the alveolus is bought into close contact with circulating blood (in the capillaries supplying the alveolus); this allows diffusion of oxygen and carbon dioxide into, and out of, the blood. Poorly oxygenated blood is supplied to the lungs, and hence to the alveolus, by the PULMONARY ARTERY; well oxygenated blood returns to the heart in the PULMONARY VEINS.

30

There are millions of alveoli within each lung and this provides an extremely large surface area for gaseous exchange. In an average-sized cat the total surface area of the alveoli is about $10m^2$, or the area covered by three double beds!

THE THORAX

The lungs lie within the thorax which protects them and plays an important role in the mechanics of breathing.

The margins or limits of the thorax are:

1. Dorsally, the thoracic vertebrae

2. Ventrally, the sternal bones (or sternebrae)

3. Laterally, the ribs (usually 13 pairs).

Each rib is composed of two parts; a dorsal bony section which articulates with (i.e. is movably joined to) a thoracic vertebra, and a more ventral section composed of cartilage. The bony and cartilaginous parts join at the costo-chondral junction (Chapter 12).

The lateral thoracic wall is composed of the ribs plus the intercostal muscles between them. In addition, muscles which arise from the thoracic vertebrae and insert onto the forelimb pass over the ribs and provide extra protection to the thorax.

4. Caudally, the diaphragm.

The diaphragm is a dome-shaped muscular and tendinous structure which separates the thorax (cranially) from the abdomen (caudally). The diaphragm has a number of small openings in it which allow the passage of various structures, e.g. the oesophagus and the aorta, from the thorax into the abdomen. A ruptured diaphragm, e.g. after a road accident, will allow abdominal contents to pass into the thorax and impede breathing.

The inner surface of the thoracic cavity (including the diaphragm) is lined by a thin layer called the pleural membrane (Fig. 6-1). This also extends over the outer surface of the lungs. There is normally a very small space between the inner and outer pleural membranes; this is called the pleural cavity. Normally the pressure within the pleural cavity is less than atmospheric pressure.

THE MECHANICS OF BREATHING

Breathing or, more correctly, pulmonary ventilation, depends upon muscular activity, and therefore requires energy. On inspiration the thorax expands in two directions;

1. Caudally, due to contraction of the diaphragm, which becomes flatter.

2. Laterally, following contraction of the intercostal muscles.

So long as the pleural cavity remains sealed expansion of the thorax causes the lungs to expand and draw air down into the alveoli.

31

All the muscles involved in breathing are of the skeletal (striated) type. If a muscle relaxant, a drug that prevents the normal function of skeletal muscle, is administered to an animal it will not be able to breathe spontaneously; in this situation ventilation MUST be assisted, either manually or by use of a mechanical respirator.

Expiration, compared with inspiration, uses very little energy. Relaxation of the diaphragm and intercostal muscles causes the thorax to become smaller; the lungs will collapse and air is forced out. Lung tissue is naturally elastic due to the presence of the protein elastin.

Under certain circumstances (e.g. following strenuous exercise) expiration may be assisted by contraction of muscles in the abdominal wall. This increases the pressure in both the abdominal and thoracic cavities, and assists the collapse of the lungs.

The alveoli are lined by an extremely thin layer of fluid which coats the epithelium and includes a substance called surfactant. Surfactant reduces the surface tension within the alveoli and helps them to expand on inspiration. In the foetus, surfactant is only produced during the last few days of pregnancy; animals born prematurely may have inadequate amounts of surfactant and this contributes to the breathing difficulties often seen in premature puppies.

DISORDERS OF BREATHING

In general, disorders of breathing may be due to:

1. A failure of air to pass into, or out of, the conducting system correctly; it is often associated with an abnormal respiratory noise.

   Examples of this problem include:

   (a) Obstruction within the lumen, e.g. a foreign body

   (b) Loss of the normal structure of the wall of the conducting tube, e.g. tracheal collapse.

   (c) Compression of the conducting tube by a mass (e.g. tumour or abscess) arising from neighbouring tissues (e.g. thyroid gland).

2. A failure of the alveoli to allow efficient gaseous exchange. Affected animals show increased respiratory effort, and may have increased respiratory rate.

   Alveoli may fail to function efficiently because of:

   (a) Reduced expansion of the lungs, due to disruption of the pleural cavity. This may follow trauma to the chest wall, disrupting the pleural cavity and allowing air to enter; this is the condition of pneumothorax. Alternatively there may be abnormal fluid (e.g. blood) in the pleural cavity, which prevents the lungs from expanding.

   (b) The presence of fluid within the alveoli, preventing the air coming into contact with the epithelium. Types of fluid include oedema (produced in heart failure) and inflammatory exudate resulting from infection (e.g. pneumonia).

CHAPTER 4:
TEMPERATURE REGULATION

We have already mentioned the link between breathing and temperature regulation in Chapter 3. This link is fundamental since the main way animals have of cooling themselves is by evaporation of water, and their main way of evaporating water is from the upper respiratory tract in panting. Not all animals pant in the obvious and special way which dogs use, but most use respiratory evaporation as a major means of cooling. This may surprise us because, as primates, we come from a group which is highly dependent on sweating and independent of panting. Horses also rely heavily on sweating. Pigs do not sweat but they get the same cooling effect by applying water externally when they wallow. Cats may get some cooling from saliva spreading. There are sweat glands in the feet of dogs and cats but their importance is minimal.

We tend to think of temperature regulation as a feature of 'warm blooded' animals, i.e. mammals and birds. But 'cold blooded' animals also control their temperature – although they do it much less precisely and almost entirely through their behaviour. Before considering the more sophisticated thermoregulation of 'warm blooded' animals it is important to emphasise that they also rely extensively on behaviour. For example if a dog feels hot it does not immediately start panting – it first moves out of the sun into shade (unless it is so fond of the sun that it stays put and pants!) If it is really hot, it sprawls on a cold surface (contacting the thinner-coated abdomen). In cold surroundings it moves to a warmer spot, curls up (and reduces its surface area for heat loss) or huddles with its owner or another dog (to reduce heat loss). Though simple, these behavioural responses are vital: the crucial difference between the dog locked in a car on a hot day and the dog lying alongside is that the latter can move into shade. (It can also pant more efficiently, but we will return to that.)

The unique achievement of birds and mammals is the precision with which they can keep temperature constant at a 'set point' well above the environmental temperature. There are regulated fluctuations in set point (e.g. rhythmic changes associated with the time of day or stage of reproductive cycle) but these differences are small. The extraordinary ability to regulate body temperature in birds and mammals depends on:

1. Being able to generate large amounts of heat chemically, internally, instead of relying on the sun (or additional physical activity) for additional warmth.
2. Being able to control both heat production and heat loss by non-behavioural, as well as behavioural means.

CO-ORDINATION OF TEMPERATURE RESPONSES

The receptors for body temperature are both deep (i.e. within the body cavities) and superficial. Deep body temperature, or core temperature, is much more tightly regulated than superficial temperature. That is quite obvious; if you go out on a cold day your skin temperature falls but your core temperature (as measured approximately by a thermometer under your tongue) does not. In fact such disparities of temperature between skin and core (e.g. rectal temperature) can be clinically important. For example, in an animal in warm surroundings they would suggest poor circulation to the skin (e.g. in shock). Normally, the superficial receptors warn the animal of what is likely to happen to core temperature if it does not take appropriate behavioural action (consciously) or trigger appropriate physiological responses (subconsiously).

Information from both deep and superficial receptors is fed to the hypothalamus, an area of the brain which is also important in regulating cardiovascular, respiratory and reproductive function. The hypothalamus co-ordinates the appropriate responses to excessive warmth or cold. It is also the site within which 'set point' is established, probably by adjusting the balance of certain chemicals. The hypothalamus is thus able to receive information concerning external temperature (from superficial receptors), core temperature (from deep body receptors), and compare the latter with 'set point'. It also measures directly the temperature of its own blood supply – another estimate of core temperature.

The remainder of this Chapter will essentially be concerned with responses controlled by the hypothalamus; those involved in the defence against heat, against cold and in the rather similar processes which lead to fever.

RESPONSE TO HEAT

The source of heat could be external or internal. The main external heat source, normally, is solar radiation. Internally the main source of additional heat would be as a by-product of muscular activity. The heat, in this case, is carried by the blood from its site of generation (muscle) to sites from which it can be lost. Mostly, in dogs, this would be the upper respiratory tract, for heat loss by evaporation of water during panting. Nevertheless, there is also substantial heat loss via increased skin blood flow, allowing the skin to become warmer and radiate heat from the animal to its environment. If the animal lies on a cool surface (or swims in cold water) there is additional heat loss from skin by conduction. The unique benefit of evaporative cooling, unlike conduction or convection, is that it works *better* as the surroundings become hotter.

The fact that evaporation of water has great cooling capacity (because substantial energy is needed to convert the liquid into vapour) is very familiar – we detect the direction of the wind by holding up a wet finger and sensing which side is cooled first by evaporation. The fact that animals rely on panting rather than sweating has the advantage that they lose pure water and no salts. It has the disadvantage that it takes muscular effort – however this additional effort is very small in dogs. Any mechanical structure, whether a bridge or a thorax, has a resonant frequency at which it is easy to make it move to and fro. Thus soldiers marching across bridges used to break step because if they were in unison and marching at the resonant frequency of the bridge, it might be so easy to set it vibrating up and down that it could disintegrate. Some of you may have seen the mechanical power of resonance in the old film of the Tacoma suspension bridge in America; a design fault allowed a gale to set it vibrating at its resonant frequency – to the extent that it collapsed. Dogs pant at the resonant frequency of their thorax thus allowing the minimum work to achieve the maximum air movement. Because the pattern of breathing is fast and shallow, there is a great increase of airflow through the upper respiratory tract (for cooling) but very little increase in alveolar air flow (leaving gas exchange virtually undisturbed – as explained in Chapter 3).

Whether animals sweat or pant, cooling is only effective if the water can evaporate. That is why 80°F (27°C) and high humidity is so much more uncomfortable than 100°F (38°C) in dry heat. New York cops have big sweat problems in summer precisely because sweat, though secreted, fails to evaporate and cool efficiently. The great benefit of air conditioning is not so much that it cools the air but that it dries the air – allowing us to cool ourselves, efficiently and comfortably.

The problem of the dog in the hot summer car is not only one of temperature and the greenhouse effect of sun through glass. If the windows are shut, the dog's panting will humidify the air (as will uncontrolled water losses through skin) and make panting less and less efficient. A bowl of water, though vital to the dog, may make this worse through further evaporation and humidification of the air – if the windows are sealed. In fact the owner who locks the dog in a sealed car defeats every means of heat loss; evaporation as already explained, radiation and conduction because the surroundings will rapidly become hotter than the dog.

RESPONSE TO COLD

Apart from the obvious – and vital – behavioural responses of finding shelter, moving towards heat, nestling into better insulation (whether a blanket or another dog) there are important physiological defences against cold. The simplest is to erect the coat thus trapping a thick layer of air – the only true biological insulator apart from fat. Erecting the coat has exactly the same effect as us putting on an additional sweater – it traps more insulating air. Incidentally, we also erect our coats in cold surroundings, but as they are so sparse, all we achieve is goose pimples!

Fat is a very effective insulator and thin animals are more vulnerable to cold, but fat has the disadvantage that it is heavy and can only be varied slowly, by removal or addition. Perhaps we should not be too disparaging about fat Labradors – they were originally fishing dogs (carrying lines between boats) and Labrador is well beyond the bikini coast. Like a polar bear, a swimming dog is only insulated by its fat as its coat no longer contains air. Nearer home, a wet coat or a wet blanket makes a sick dog much more vulnerable to cold. And of course newborn animals are especially vulnerable until their mothers lick them dry.

We have all heard of people 'blue with cold', though I doubt if we have seen many! Why blue? Because we respond by reducing skin blood flow, especially to the extremities (ears, fingers, toes) and reduced blood flow, combined with continuing oxygen consumption by tissues leads to cyanosis (Chapter 3).

So far the responses to cold have not involved increased use (waste) of energy, just reduced losses (like double glazing and loft insulation). For every animal, however, there is an environmental temperature ('critical temperature') below which it can only maintain its body temperature by using more energy. Above this temperature, room heating is probably a waste of money (especially in a farm animal). But below it, the animal is actually using some of the energy available from food to preserve body temperature. It may not be uncomfortable nor in danger – but if it is a farm animal, it is wasting food – converting it into heat instead of meat. A young or thin animal has a higher critical temperature, i.e. needs warmer surroundings to avoid 'burning' its own energy. So does a sick animal.

Energy can be applied to heat production in two ways.

(a) As a by-product of movement; cold animals tense their muscles, move about more actively and, ultimately, they shiver, i.e. move muscles to generate heat.

(b) Directly through metabolism. Hormones can increase the rate at which the various biochemical reactions in the body generate heat. This is particularly true of those in liver and muscle (quite apart from shivering). Naturally this uses reserves of fat or carbohydrate (unless food intake increases in the longer term). Young animals especially have a particular fat ('brown fat') which is not just an energy reserve but highly adapted for heat generation and can also localise it to the vicinity of certain blood supplies.

Given insulation, food and good health, warm blooded animals can resist extremely low temperatures, provided their tissues are not frozen and thereby damaged. The main factors undermining temperature regulation are disruption of insulation (by rain or wind), lack of food, shelter, or freedom to find them, and disease or anaesthesia.

ABNORMALITIES OF TEMPERATURE REGULATION

The most important disturbance, clinically, is fever because we use the rise of temperature for diagnosis of infection (though it is not foolproof). It is not, however, a failure of temperature regulation. When you begin to have 'flu you feel cold and shiver – just as if you really were cold. You even restrict your skin blood flow and look pale. That is because, in the hypothalamus, the regulatory set point is increased during fever. Normal body temperature therefore feels cold and the animal responds exactly as it would to genuine cold (birds fluff up their feathers, tuck their head under a wing, etc.). When the fever subsides, it is because set point returns to normal. The febrile temperature now feels too hot and the animal responds as if to genuine heat until these responses return the temperature to normal (in your case you will be flushed and sweating at this stage). The magic of aspirin and similar drugs is that they return an elevated (febrile) set point to normal but do not depress a normal set point.

Simply cooling a febrile animal will not help it in the least – it will merely use all its regulatory responses including shivering, to regain the higher temperature so long as fever elevates its set point. On the other hand an animal with heat stroke urgently needs to be cooled because its temperature is rising *despite* its regulatory responses – they have been overwhelmed.

In fact fever does not usually take body temperature up to dangerous levels – even before antibacterial drugs – and on balance it is probably beneficial in the animal's fight against infection. Surprisingly, cold blooded animals show fever during infection – provided you allow them the chance to increase their temperature in the only way possible, through the behavioural choice of warmer surroundings. Even fish and insects can be febrile! Fever itself is achieved by a hormone released from white blood cells during infection (and in some other circumstances) and reaching the hypothalamus to elevate its set point. Precisely the same hormone acts in all animals – from scorpions to people.

Newborn animals are vulnerable to disturbances of body temperature, especially cooling, because they have less fat reserves and insulation, more restricted behavioural choices, and their thermoregulatory mechanisms may not yet be fully effective (including fever – which can also be suppressed by malnutrition). In addition, because they are small, they have a relatively big area for heat loss and a relatively small volume within which to generate heat. (Desert animals tend to be small; ice ages produce woolly mammoths). If you consider the material needed to make a cube, the area of each face only increases with the length squared, whereas the enclosed volume increases with the length cubed. Big objects, including animals, have a bigger volume per surface area.

Anaesthesia can undermine body temperature both by depressing the regulatory centres, interfering with the distribution of blood flow, and restricting behavioural and muscular responses to cold. Shock has similar or additional effects so that it is necessary to ensure that body temperature does not fall. Excessive warming, however, would be counterproductive; it would open up skin bloodflow (to shed heat) and undermine the protection of blood pressure (Chapter 6). Finally, and most obviously, the veterinary nurse can undermine the animal's thermoregulation if she administers substantial volumes of life-saving fluid therapy – but forgets to warm the fluids to something near body temperature.

CHAPTER 5:
BLOOD AND TISSUE FLUIDS

If you weigh around 8 stone (50 kg), about 30 kg (l) of it (6½ gallons) is simply water; 60% of bodyweight. In a young or very thin animal, the percentage is higher, in an old or fat animal it would be less, simply because fat deposits contain little water. Blood is so important that you could imagine that it accounted for a larger proportion of body water but it actually makes up rather less than 10% of bodyweight. Most of the body water (⅔) is inside the cells (intracellular fluid, ICF; Fig. 5-1). The remaining ⅓ (20% of bodyweight) is outside cells and is therefore called extracellular fluid (ECF) – extra in the sense of outside (as in extraterrestrial), not spare or additional.

You might think that blood was part of ECF but it consists of cells, both red and white, suspended in the liquid plasma. Only the plasma is part of ECF and, suprisingly, it makes up merely ¼ of its volume (5% of bodyweight; Fig. 5-1). The rest of the ECF is the interstitial fluid, filling the tissue spaces around the capillaries and between the cells. This interstitial fluid, or tissue fluid, provides a constant environment for the cells, supplying their needs and removing their waste; to do this it is constantly replenished from plasma, by exchange across the thin walls of the capillary blood vessels.

ECF and ICF

Plasma and interstitial fluid (both ECF) are rich in sodium (Na^+) whereas ICF is rich in potassium (K^+). This difference is maintained by sodium-potassium 'pumps' in cell membranes; sodium leaks into cells but is constantly pumped out so that its concentration is low in ICF, high in ECF. As sodium is expelled, potassium enters so that ICF is rich in K^+ whereas ECF K^+ concentration is low. The pumps need energy; they use ATP.

If cells are in areas with poor blood supply, or their energy metabolism is depressed, or if their membranes are damaged, they will fail to accumulate potassium properly, or it will leak out. Since ICF is twice the volume of ECF and contains 40 times the K^+ concentration, small losses of ICF K^+ can produce dangerous rises in ECF K^+ concentration. For example, a rise from

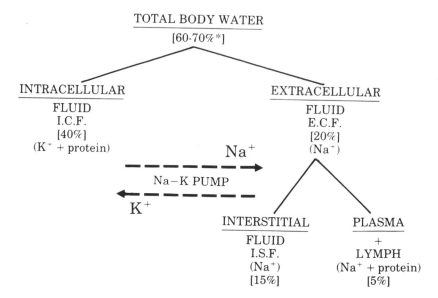

[%] = litres of fluid /100 kg body weight
( ) = main osmotic solute

TOTAL BODY WATER
[60-70%*]

INTRACELLULAR
FLUID
I.C.F.
[40%]
(K⁺ + protein)

Na⁺

Na–K PUMP

K⁺

EXTRACELLULAR
FLUID
E.C.F.
[20%]
(Na⁺)

INTERSTITIAL
FLUID
I.S.F.
(Na⁺)
[15%]

PLASMA
+
LYMPH
(Na⁺ + protein)
[5%]

* More if young, less if fat/old.

Figure 5-1. Distribution of body water.

the normal value (4-5 mmol/l) to 7-8 mmol/l is liable to disrupt heart function; a pound of muscle contains the necessary amount of potassium if it were all lost at once. The event is unlikely but the fact that a pound of hamburger contains a lethal dose of K^+ (not when you eat it!) emphasises the importance of intracellular K^+. Although the ECF concentration of K^+ is low, it must not fall too far below normal; at 2-3 mmol/l the reduction would depress muscle function (Chapter 12).

It is equally important that sodium is kept out of cells. When two solutions are separated by a membrane in the body, water tends to flow freely from the one with the lower total concentration (i.e. of all dissolved contents or 'solutes') to the one with the higher concentration. This tendency of water to diffuse between solutions in such a way as to equalise their solute concentration is called 'osmosis'. The concentration which dictates osmotic water movement is the total number of chemical particles (ions or molecules) in the solution, regardless of their weight. A litre of water with 180 mg of glucose has the same osmotic concentration as one with only 30mg of salt. This is because each molecule of glucose weighs three times as much as a salt molecule and each salt molecule yields two dissolved particles, a sodium ion (Na^+) and a chloride ion (Cl^-). Now ICF is rich in a variety of solutes apart from K^+, so in order for ECF to exist, to avoid having its water sucked into cells by osmosis, it must contain solutes to resist this tendency otherwise ECF volume would shrink and cells would swell. The main solutes of ECF are sodium (140-150

40

mmol/l) and chloride (100 mmol/l). It is the sodium pump which keeps sodium (and therefore the associated chloride) in ECF and thereby enables it to maintain its volume; sodium is the osmotic skeleton of extracellular fluid. Finally, although sodium and potassium have the same positive electrical charge, the pump expels more sodium than the potassium which it brings in. The outside of the cell membrane therefore becomes positively charged and the inside becomes more negative. This voltage, this potential difference, is exactly the same in character as that between the '+' and '−' terminals of a torch battery, simply about twenty times smaller. It is extremely important in cells such as nerve and muscle because it makes them electrically 'excitable' (Chapter 10). In special circumstances (e.g. electric eels) 'batteries' of cells can generate very large voltages indeed.

UNITS OF MEASUREMENT

Already we have started to use some curious units of measurement, mmol/l, though you may have seen them on fluid therapy packs. Since movement of water by osmosis depends on numbers of particles rather than their weight, we need a unit of measurement which reflects this. We obtain such a unit by 'correcting' for the different weights of different ions or molecules, i.e. by dividing the weight of a solute by its molecular weight or formula weight. The molecular weight of glucose is 180; if we have the molecular weight in milligrams (180 mg) we have one millimole (mmol). If we have a millimole of salt (59 mg) we obtain a solution containing a millimole each of sodium (23 mg) and chloride (36 mg). If the volume of the solution is one litre we have 1 mmol/l each of sodium chloride, Na^+ and Cl^-. Because the 1 mmol/l of sodium and of chloride each exert an osmotic effect (i.e. 2 m osmoles/l, = 2 mOsm/l) we would need 2 mmol/l of glucose to produce the same osmotic concentration. Solutions with the same osmotic effect as normal plasma are **'isotonic'**. If they are more concentrated, they are **hypertonic** (and will draw fluid out of cells). If they are more dilute they are **hypotonic** (and will yield water to cells, making them swell).

TISSUE FLUID AND PLASMA

We already know that tissue fluid, interstitial fluid, needs constant replenishment from plasma. How does this occur? In effect, there is another circulatory system outside the blood vessels, in the tissue spaces. It is illustrated in Fig. 5-2.

At the arterial end of the capillary water and solutes are driven into interstitial fluid by the hydrostatic pressure inside the capillary. (Hydrostatic pressure simply means pressure in a liquid resulting from its own weight or pressure applied to it). At the venous end of the capillary, hydrostatic pressure has fallen because of the reduced fluid volume of fluid remaining inside. In the absence of this outward force, water is retrieved from interstitial fluid into plasma, drawn by the osmotic effect of the plasma proteins. Water and solutes can thus circulate in and out of interstitial fluid, from plasma and back again.

Obviously this system only works because the protein concentration in plasma is much higher than in interstitial fluid. This in turn depends on the

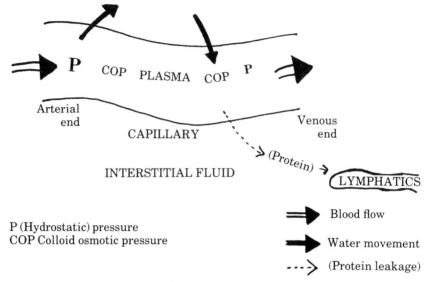

P (Hydrostatic) pressure
COP Colloid osmotic pressure

Blood flow

Water movement

(Protein leakage)

Figure 5-2. Capillary exchange.

ability of the capillaries to retain solutes about the size of albumin or larger; smaller solutes escape into interstitial fluid. Since albumin has a smaller molecule than globulin it is the more important of the two main plasma proteins, from an osmotic point of view; a given weight contains more particles of solute. If protein should spill into interstitial fluid, either from damaged capillaries or cells, the excess is swept away by the lymphatics, ultimately returning to circulation. The lymphatics have other important functions, in defence against disease and transport of digested fat but where body fluids are concerned, their paramount function is to keep the concentration of interstitial protein low. When the latter begins to rise, lymphatic flow increases thus removing the excess.

Disturbances of the system for fluid exchange across capillaries can result in accumulation of excess interstitial fluid. This is called **oedema** and can result in visible or even dramatic puffy swelling. There are several causes and they are predictable from what you have already read.

1. Too much protein in interstitial fluid; blocked lymphatic drainage or leaky (damaged) capillaries – e.g. allergy or burns.

2. Not enough protein in plasma; failure to synthesise sufficient albumin in the liver or loss of plasma protein from damaged gut or kidney. Malnutrition, if severe, can also cause this.

3. Too high a pressure within the capillaries. This can occur because the arterioles are too relaxed as a result of warmth or allergy. More usually it is because venous pressure is too high

   a) because the heart is failing to pump the blood onwards efficiently, or

   b) because of obstruction or direct pressure affecting veins, e.g. clots (thrombi), external pressure from tight bandages or casts.

Both in veins and lymphatics movement of surrounding muscle helps propulsion of the contained fluid and valves ensure that it moves only in the correct direction, i.e. from the tissues towards the heart. Inactivity therefore predisposes to oedema. Thus our feet swell in hot weather (arteriolar dilation) and on long bus journeys (inactivity plus pressure on leg veins).

Tissue oedema is unsightly but not life-threatening. Similar processes leading to oedema formation within the abdominal cavity lead to the accumulation of free fluid (ascites), often sufficient to distend the abdomen. Such accumulations, if severe, will impair movement of the diaphragm and increase the work of breathing. Ascites often indicates underlying heart failure or liver disease, for the reasons just described. Malnutrition can also cause ascites and a pot-bellied abdomen – though it has to be severe and other factors are then involved. The one form of oedema (other than brain oedema) which is potentially fatal is pulmonary oedema. The usual cause is heart failure, often temporarily induced by overload with intravenous fluids, probably because they have been given too fast rather than too generously. Dilution of plasma albumin is often blamed for pulmonary oedema but it is a minor factor.

Apart from carrying the red and white blood cells in suspension, plasma also carries many important chemicals in solution. These include:

1. Mineral salts (yielding ions such as Na^+, K^+, Ca^{++}, bicarbonate, etc.).

2. Nutrients (glucose, amino acids, fatty acids, vitamins).

3. Waste products (urea, creatinine).

4. Hormones, which regulate cell function.

5. Proteins

    (a) Albumin – which retrieves fluid from tissue spaces (see above) and also binds and carries minerals (e.g. Ca^{++}).

    (b) Other proteins which bind and carry minerals and hormones.

    (c) Globulins which help protect against infection.

    (d) Clotting factors (see below).

Blood also carries particles (**platelets**) derived from cells which are important in sealing wounds and in clotting.

CLOTTING OF BLOOD

The first defence of a wounded blood vessel against blood loss (haemorrhage) precedes clotting. The vessel retracts if it has been cut through, and the rougher the damage, the better the retraction – hence 'clean' cuts bleed freely. The next stages of the defence against haemorrhage is that platelets adhere to the damaged surface of the vessel and aggregate to form a seal. This is particularly effective against minor damage and prevents many everyday wear and tear injuries from bleeding; its importance becomes obvious when platelet number or function is defective and extensive minute haemorrhages appear (petechiae). Platelets also produce an enzyme which is one of the

43

factors able to trigger clotting – hence they are also called thrombocytes (a thrombus is a clot). The entire defence against haemorrhage (of which the formation and hardening of a clot is the final stage) is called 'haemostasis'.

Basically clotting is simple. Blood contains a protein (fibrinogen) made in the liver (Fig. 5-3). In suitable circumstances it turns into fibrin, which is no longer soluble, and forms a fibrous mesh which traps blood cells. The clot, once formed, retracts (this causes a better seal and squeezes serum out). The clot then hardens (and becomes a scab). Both retraction and hardening (stabilisation) are brought about by platelets. Because clotting is such a crucial defence yet has the potential to be so dangerous, blocking vessels completely as in **thrombosis,** the control system is very complicated.

Essentially it is a dual control involving 'extrinsic' and 'intrinsic' systems. The intrinsic system (Fig. 5-3) is rather slow and depends on contact damage to blood; this is what allows blood to clot in syringes, glassware, or wherever it contacts a strange or damaged surface. Such surfaces can be prevented from

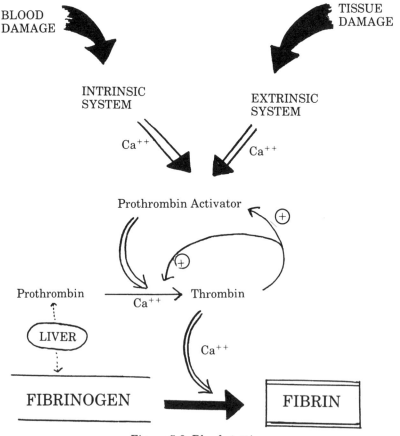

Figure 5-3. Blood clotting.

44

causing damaging contact by a silicone coating. Tissue damage accelerates clotting by triggering the extrinsic system. Both, through various steps, cause the liberation in blood of prothrombin activator, but need calcium to do so. Prothrombin activator is an enzyme which triggers rapid conversion of prothrombin, a plasma protein produced in the liver, to thrombin, again a step which needs calcium. It is thrombin which converts fibrinogen, another plasma protein made in the liver, to fibrin and yet again, calcium is needed.

This 'cascade' of reactions, once triggered, accelerates explosively, hence the rapidity of clotting. Partly this results from 'positive feedback' (Chapter 1) with thrombin, once formed, accelerating the production of its precursors (prothrombin activator and prothrombin) thus accelerating its own production.

Obviously with so many steps dependent on calcium, clotting can be blocked by chemicals such as citrate, oxalate and EDTA which prevent calcium from being active in plasma, by combining with it. Such chemicals are used to prevent blood samples from clotting ('anti-coagulants'). Heparin, another anticoagulant, is normally produced in the body by 'mast cells', especially in the lungs and liver. It protects them from further growth of any clots which they receive and works by inhibiting both prothrombin activator and thrombin. The lungs also contain enzymes to break down circulating clots ('fibrinolysis') because while an attached clot may be life-saving by preventing haemorrhage, a detached clot (or embolus) in circulation can lodge in a vital blood vessel and block it.

What stops a protective clot from growing right along a blood vessel or blocking it completely? The further you go from the point of injury, the more the blood flow dilutes the trigger factors and therefore the less the effectiveness of clotting. The important implication is that poor or stagnant blood flow will increase the risk of extensive and dangerous clotting from trivial injury; this is the problem of old people, inactive during prolonged bed rest.

The liver is important in producing clotting precursors so liver disease, if severe, may lead to the risk of haemorrhage. Perhaps the worst example of defective clotting in dogs and cats comes from warfarin poisoning. The lethal effect is to interfere with any clotting by preventing prothrombin production and to simultaneously produce capillary damage; this combination obviously produces severe and extensive haemorrhage. The treatment with vitamin K reflects the fact that it is normally involved in prothrombin production but warfarin interferes with its action. A hereditary deficiency of clotting factors, haemophilia, occurs in dogs and cats as it does in man, though fortunately it is rare; it leaves the victim susceptible to lethal haemorrhage, even from minor injury.

If, instead of using an anticoagulant, we allow a blood sample to clot, the clot eventually retracts and is seen as a compact mass in a clear straw-coloured liquid which is serum. It differs from plasma only in that the clotting factors have been consumed (fibrinogen, prothrombin, etc.).

45

PCV: ANAEMIA

The proportion of a blood sample occupied by cells and plasma can be determined by centrifuging it in a glass capillary tube. The centrifugal force packs the cells against the sealed end as a red column leaving the clear plasma entirely separated. The percentage of blood volume occupied by the cells (mostly RBC) is thus easily measured (**packed cell volume, PCV,** or **haematocrit**). This measurement will be low where a lack of RBC has caused anaemia or where haemorrhage has been severe. Haemorrhage does not directly depress PCV because both red cells and plasma are lost but the physiological response to haemorrhage transfers interstitial fluid back into circulation (Chapter 6). This 'haemodilution' reduces the PCV. Lack of RBC is one cause of **anaemia** but basically it is a lack of haemoglobin and can also arise, therefore, from failure to produce sufficient haemoglobin in otherwise normal RBC.

BLOOD CELLS (Fig. 5-4)

The function of the most plentiful components, the RBC and platelets, have already been described and the latter are cell derivatives, no longer true cells. Both are continuously produced in the bone marrow. The RBC are destroyed in liver, spleen and bone marrow after a life of about 3-4 months. The young RBC, like all other cells, have nuclei but (except in birds) the nucleus disappears before the mature RBC enters circulation.

The division of white cells (WBC) or 'leukocytes' into granulocytes or agranulocytes simply describes whether or not they contain visible granules when stained under the microscope. Those that do are further classified according to whether the granules stain with basic, neutral or acidic dyes such as eosin. The neutrophils tend to have nuclei of various shapes (multiple lobes) hence the name 'polymorphs'. Their important role is to move into damaged tissue and engulf bacteria or debris, i.e. they act as **phagocytes.** Appropriately, infected animals produce far more neutrophils and this can be detected when cells are differentially counted in a blood smear. Neutrophils are not the only phagocytes; they are helped by large agranulocytes called monocytes, or macrophages. Obviously these scavenger cells will be found in tissues, as well as blood. They not only destroy invading bacteria, they help to identify them as targets for the lymphocytes.

The lymphocytes play two crucial roles in the defence against infection (**immunity**). They respond to alien proteins – usually on the surface of bacteria or viruses – by proliferating and either

1. Producing antibodies ('**humoral immunity**'); 'B cells', or

2. Acting as killer cells, or as helper cells (which help B cells or macrophages to function more effectively). These 'T cells' thus have multiple functions in producing **cellular immunity.**

Cellular or humoral immunity is not only the basis of resistance to disease but can also produce it through allergy, hypersensitivity, rejection (e.g. of alien blood transfusions) or even autoimmunity – confusing 'self' cells with alien cells and attacking them.

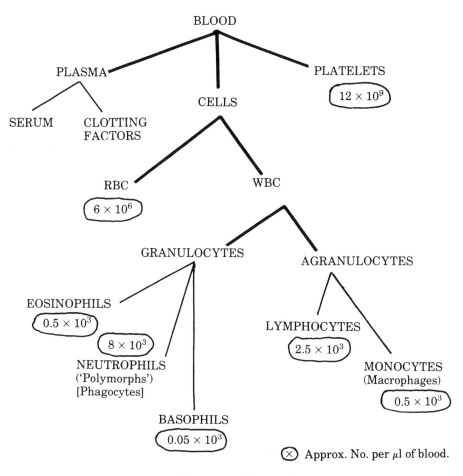

Figure 5-4. Blood cells.

Both tissue cells and red cells can be 'typed' according to their immune compatability with those of other individuals. This is the basis of matching of blood types for transfusion or organ types for transplantation. Since the peak production of antibodies takes 10 days or so, a first transfusion of mismatched blood may be harmless – but a second transfusion will be damaged by the waiting antibodies. Unfortunately, if a bitch has formed antibodies to a mismatched transfusion she may pass these to her puppies through colostrum (first milk) and, depending on their blood type, their own RBC may be attacked.

Eosinophils are especially involved in the response to parasites and in allergic reactions. The basophils (including 'mast cells') are the least plentiful WBC and they produce heparin (already mentioned) and a number of substances involved in inflammation and allergy, including histamine.

47

Essentially all the white cells share a common function; they respond to foreign proteins. Usually this response is defensive (immunity) but sometimes it is more harmful than the protein against which it is directed, as in allergy or hypersensitivity. Immunity, as already discussed, can be humoral or cellular in mechanism and it can be active (where the animal responds for itself to the foreign protein or **'antigen'**) or passive where the animal receives ready made antibodies, either in colostrum or by injection. Most vaccines inject antigen, suitably treated to still be able to arouse an antibody response but not to cause disease. Injection of antibodies produces immediate protection but it is short-lived because the injected antibodies are broken down and the animal's lymphocytes, not having 'seen' the antigen do not 'know' how to produce more. The boosting of immunity by vaccines and its suppression to permit transplantation has become the clinical aspect of an entire branch of medicine – immunology – which is essentially the study of the activities of white blood cells, both protective and harmful. Thanks to biotechnology, it is becoming possible to 'instruct' bacterial 'factories' to produce antigens which can stimulate immunity but are incapable of causing disease; these will be the basis of safer vaccines, many of them allowing multiple protection against a variety of diseases.

CHAPTER 6:
CIRCULATORY SYSTEM

ANATOMY OF THE CIRCULATORY SYSTEM

The components of the circulatory system are:

(a) **The heart,** a muscular pump situated in the chest which supplies blood, under pressure to the arteries.

(b) **The arteries** are a branching system of blood vessels which deliver blood to

(c) **The capillary beds** within the tissues of the body.

(d) The collecting system of vessels, **the veins,** carries blood from the tissues back to the heart.

(e) **The lymphatics** return any excess tissue fluid (lost from capillaries) to the main veins.

The control systems which enable the system to work efficiently and respond to changing bodily needs will be described but first we need to consider the structure of the different components and relate it to their function.

THE HEART

The heart is a muscular organ situated in the thorax where it lies within the mediastinum. The mediastinum is the central section of the thoracic cavity which lies between the left and right pleural cavities (Fig. 6-1). The outer surface of the heart is covered by a translucent membrane called the pericardium. The heart is normally cone-shaped, with a distinct "apex" which is positioned ventrally next to the sternum, and a broader "base" situated more dorsally in the chest (Fig. 6-3). Notice that the base of the heart is **above** its apex.

Superficial examination of the heart reveals numerous large blood vessels entering and leaving the heart. On closer examination one sees, in addition, smaller blood vessels running in distinct "grooves" on the surface of the

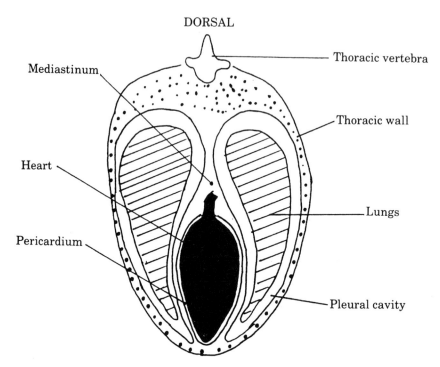

DORSAL

Mediastinum

Thoracic vertebra

Thoracic wall

Heart

Lungs

Pericardium

Pleural cavity

Figure 6-1. Diagrammatic cross-section of the thorax to demonstrate the position of the heart.

heart; these are the coronary arteries responsible for supplying blood to the heart muscle. So the heart does not 'use' the blood which it contains: it uses blood supplied by the coronary arteries, which arise from the aorta.

Internally, the left and right side of the heart each possess an atrium (collecting chamber) and a ventricle (pumping chamber) (Fig. 6-2). The wall of the heart (myocardium) is composed of cardiac muscle, which is a special type of muscle (Chapter 12). The right side of the heart pumps blood into the pulmonary circulation (to the lungs), whereas the left side serves the systemic circulation (to the rest of the body). The difference in arterial blood pressure between these two circulatory systems is reflected in the thickness of the myocardium: that surrounding the left ventricle is up to five times thicker than that of the right ventricle. The left and right sides of the heart are not exactly aligned with the left and right sides of the body; during embryonic development the heart twists to the left so that its left side faces somewhat caudally, its right side rather cranially.

Within the heart blood normally flows from the atrium through a valve (called the atrio-ventricular valve) into the ventricle. The atrio-ventricular valves prevent blood flowing from the ventricle back into the atrium during systole (the period of ventricular contraction). Because of the high pressures encountered in the ventricles during systole there is a risk that the flaps of the

50

valve could be "blown open" allowing backflow of blood. To prevent this the valve flaps are attached by fibrous strands (called chordae tendinae) to the papillary muscles which project from the ventricular wall (Fig. 6-2). They function like the guy-ropes and pegs used to hold a tent in position in high winds.

To understand the structure of the heart more clearly, one can follow the passage of blood through its chambers. During the resting phase, or diastole, venous blood flows into the right atrium. Once it is full, the right atrio-ventricular valve opens allowing blood to pass into the right ventricle. During systole the ventricle contracts, the atrio-ventricular valve closes, and blood is pumped into the pulmonary artery. Lying in the wall of the artery is a small valve, the pulmonic valve, which is forced open during systole, but closes during diastole. This prevents backflow into the ventricle, and helps

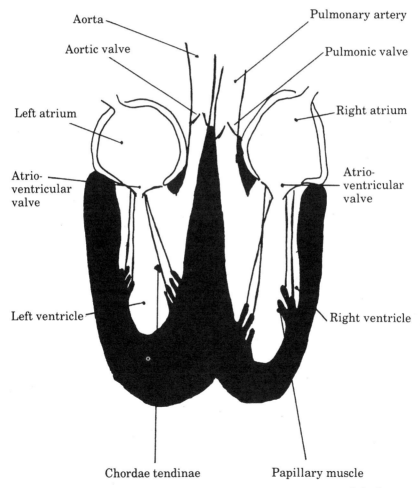

Figure 6-2. Diagram to demonstrate the internal structure of the heart.

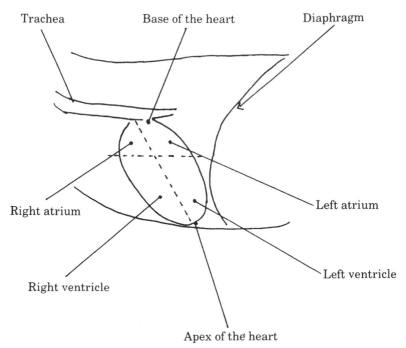

Trachea   Base of the heart   Diaphragm

Right atrium   Left atrium

Right ventricle   Left ventricle

Apex of the heart

Figure 6-3. Diagram to show the appearance of the heart on a normal lateral chest radiograph.

maintain the pulmonary arterial blood pressure. Blood returns from the lungs in the pulmonary veins which enter the left atrium. The left atrio-ventricular valve opens allowing blood to pass into the left ventricle, from where it is pumped out under high pressure into the aorta. The aortic valve lies in the wall of the aorta and serves a similar role to the pulmonic valve, preventing backflow of blood and maintaining arterial pressure. The left and right atria contract simultaneously, as do the two ventricles.

Having considered the internal and external structure of the heart one might question the relevance of all this knowledge. One only sees the heart in a living animal at the time of thoracotomy (surgical exposure of the thoracic contents), which is not commonly performed in veterinary practice. However, we do observe the living heart or, more correctly, its image, on a chest radiograph. From a knowledge of basic cardiac anatomy it is possible to identify (approximately) the various chambers of the heart: on a lateral chest radiograph a line drawn from the base of the heart to its apex divides the heart into the more cranially positioned right side and the more caudally positioned left side. The atria are positioned dorsal to the ventricles (Fig. 6-3).

The inherent orderly contraction of the myocardium relies upon an internal conducting system, composed of specialised muscle cells. The major pacemaker of the heart is the sino-atrial (SA) node which lies in the wall of the right atrium. There is a second trigger region, the atrio-ventricular (A-V) node lying in the myocardium, between the left and right atria (Fig. 6-4).

Leading from the AV node is a bundle of conducting tissue which runs through the wall of the ventricles, and is responsible for conducting nervous impulses to this chamber.

Autonomic nerves within the thorax pass to the sino-atrial node where they influence the rate of electrical activity. Stimulation of sympathetic nerves accelerates the heart rate; this is called tachycardia. In contrast, the parasympathetic nerves (from the vagus nerve) cause a slowing of the heart rate; this is called bradycardia.

DEVELOPMENT OF THE HEART

Within the embryo, the heart develops from a primitive tube which later is divided into the different sections already described. The atria develop from one chamber which becomes divided by a septum (or dividing layer). Initially there is a hole in the septum allowing blood to pass between the right and left sides of the circulatory systems. At birth, the hole closes, effectively

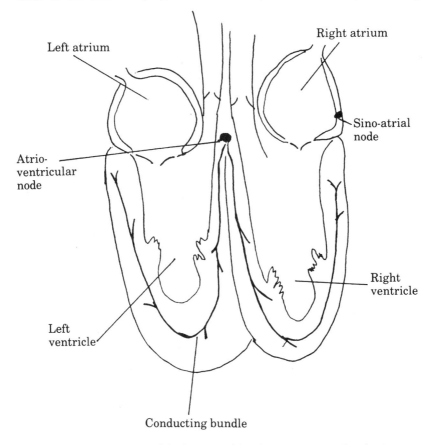

Figure 6-4. Cross-section of the heart to show the intrinsic conduction system.

53

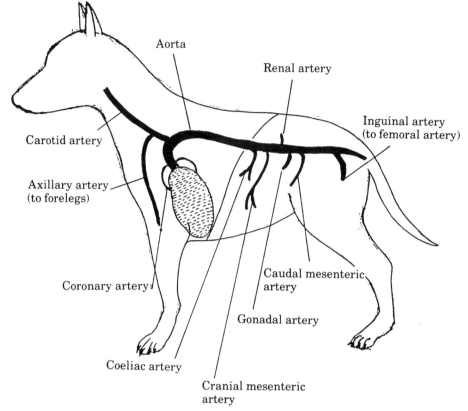

Aorta

Renal artery

Inguinal artery
(to femoral artery)

Carotid artery

Axillary artery
(to forelegs)

Coronary artery

Caudal mesenteric
artery

Gonadal artery

Coeliac artery

Cranial mesenteric
artery

Figure 6-5. Longitudinal section of the body to demonstrate the aorta, and its major branches.

separating the two circulatory systems. Similarly, the ventricles develop from one chamber which becomes divided by the interventricular septum before birth. In some animals these septae may fail to form correctly, causing a congenital defect (i.e. one that is present at birth). There is mixing of blood from the systemic and pulmonary circulations which may lead to production of a cardiac "murmur" due to turbulent blood flow.

In the foetus, the lungs serve no role in gaseous exchange which, instead, occurs at the placenta. Hence, blood in the pulmonary artery is diverted into the aorta, along a small vessel, the ductus arteriosus. At birth, this vessel closes, ensuring separation of the right and left sides of the circulation. Failure of closure leads to the condition of "patent ductus arteriosus", which is usually associated with a "murmur" due to turbulence of blood flowing from the high pressure aorta into the pulmonary artery.

THE ARTERIES

Arteries are thick-walled blood vessels which carry blood under high pressure away from the heart. This blood is well oxygenated, EXCEPT for the PULMONARY ARTERY which carries poorly oxygenated blood to the lungs.

54

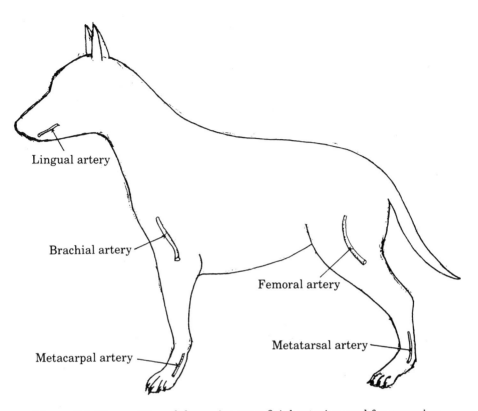

Lingual artery

Brachial artery

Femoral artery

Metacarpal artery

Metatarsal artery

Figure 6-6. The position of the major superficial arteries used for assessing the peripheral pulse.

Blood is pumped from the left ventricle into the aorta, and the first branches from this are the coronary arteries, supplying blood to the myocardium itself. However, due to compression during contraction of the surrounding myocardium, blood only flows through the coronary arteries during diastole. The next branches of the aorta are the arteries serving the head, neck and forelimbs. The aorta continues caudally within the chest, passing through the diaphragm, to run dorsally in the abdomen (Fig. 6-5). Along its course it gives off more branches which supply the organs of the abdomen and pelvis, before dividing in the caudal abdomen to provide the arterial supply to the hindlimbs. The names given to the arteries (and veins) of the body are often the cause of much consternation; there is, however, no need for this! The naming of the major blood vessels is, in most cases, quite logical, taking their name either from structures close to them (e.g. the femoral artery running close to the femur) or from the organ which they supply (e.g. the hepatic artery supplies the liver, the renal artery supplies the kidney).

Within the tissues of the body arteries rarely reach their termination without initially giving off side branches (or collateral vessels). Hence, a volume of tissue may be supplied with blood from a number of small arteries which link up (or anastomose) with each other. This is an efficient safety mechanism which ensures that if one branch is occluded then there will not be instant necrosis (cell death) in that region. In fact, the collateral vessels will dilate to ensure that total blood flow to the region is not reduced. A good example of the importance of collateral circulation comes from the fact that ligation of the femoral artery does not lead to instant death of the leg, thanks to the collateral supply which runs through the muscles of the thigh. Unfortunately certain tissues have a poorly developed collateral circulation; here, if an end-artery is occluded, the area of tissue that it supplies rapidly dies. A poor collateral circulation is seen in certain areas of the brain, and in the coronary arteries; this explains why a blood clot (thrombus) in these arteries can have such serious clinical effects, as seen in cases of coronary thrombosis or "heart attack" in people. (An area of dead tissue due to interruption of blood supply is an 'infarct'; tissue death is 'necrosis'.)

At certain sites within the body, arteries run close enough to the overlying skin to be palpated. It is possible to monitor the peripheral arterial pulse at these sites, allowing assessment of its rate and strength. The sites commonly used are:

1. **Femoral artery;** on the inner (medial) surface of the thigh.

2. **Brachial artery;** on the medial surface of the forelimb, proximal to the elbow joint.

3. The **metacarpal arteries;** on the palmar surface of the metacarpal region of the forelimb, and

4. The **metatarsal arteries;** on the plantar surface of the metatarsal region of the hindlimb.

5. The **lingual artery,** on the ventral surface of the tongue; this is only accessible in the anaesthetised patient (Fig. 6-6).

The ability to locate these arteries (in both the dog and cat) is an important clinical skill, allowing you to monitor the cardiovascular system in both conscious and anaesthetised patients.

The carotid arteries pass up the neck, on either side of the trachea, supplying blood to the head, neck and, most important of all, to the brain. Positioned in the wall of the aorta and the carotid arteries are two types of receptors which monitor the blood flowing to the brain. Baroreceptors monitor arterial blood pressure whereas chemoreceptors monitor the chemical composition (pO_2, pCO_2 and pH) of the blood. Afferent (i.e. sensory) nerves pass from these receptors along the neck to the brain. (We will encounter different chemoreceptors when we consider taste and smell, Chapter 11).

THE VEINS

The veins are thin-walled vessels which serve to transport blood from the capillaries of the various tissues back to the heart. They normally carry poorly oxygenated blood, EXCEPT for the PULMONARY VEIN which carries well-oxygenated blood from the lungs to the left atrium. Veins also act as a reservoir for blood, and their volume can be increased or decreased by relaxation or contraction of smooth muscle in their wall. There is no distinct pump attached to the venous system, so this begs the question of how does blood flow back to the heart? Contraction and relaxation of the surrounding skeletal muscles compresses the thin-walled veins and causes blood to flow. To ensure blood only flows towards the heart there is a series of valves in the wall of the veins. The importance of the muscular "pump" in producing venous blood flow is highlighted in soldiers who stand for long periods "on parade". There is little activity of the leg muscles, leading to reduced venous return and this can lead to a soldier actually fainting! Experienced soldiers are aware of the problem and know that regular contraction and relaxation of the leg muscles (without actually moving their legs!) will prevent this problem.

Blood flow within veins is easily stopped by applying external pressure to the vessel. This is the basis of "raising a vein" for an intravenous injection, where a superficial vein is temporarily occluded. Similarly, pressure exerted on a vein by surrounding tissues, with prolonged occlusion of blood flow, leads to a rise in the pressure within the venules and capillaries. This explains why a tight bandage applied to a dog's forearm leads to swelling and oedema of the forepaw.

The distribution of veins within the body to a large extent mirrors that of the arteries, with veins and arteries often running side-by-side. Similarly, there is usually collateral venous drainage from the body's tissues; in the limbs this is achieved by there being a deep (close to the bones) and superficial (close to the skin) system of veins. In the abdomen, blood draining from the intestines and stomach flows in a serious of veins directly to the liver; this is called the hepatic portal venous system and is discussed in more detail in Chapter 8.

The two veins returning blood to the right atrium are the cranial vena cava (blood from the head, neck and forelimbs) and the caudal vena cava (blood from the abdomen and hindlimbs).

The commonest route by which veterinary surgeons gain access to the blood system of an animal (be it for intravenous administration of drugs or to obtain a blood sample for laboratory examination) is by making use of one of the superficial veins (Fig. 6-7). Those commonly used are:

1. **Cephalic vein;** running on the cranial surface of the forearm, and occluded by applying pressure at the elbow joint.

2. **Lateral saphenous vein;** running on the lateral surface of the tibia and Achilles tendon. It is quite mobile with respect to surrounding tissues, a feature which can make intravenous injection difficult. This vein is occluded by applying pressure over the caudal surface of the stifle.

3. **Jugular vein;** drains blood from the head and neck, and runs just lateral to the trachea. Pressure applied at the base of the neck will occlude blood flow in this vein.

4. **Lingual vein;** runs on the ventral surface of the tongue, next to the lingual artery. It can only be used in the anaesthetised patient, and pressure is applied at the base of the tongue to occlude blood flow.

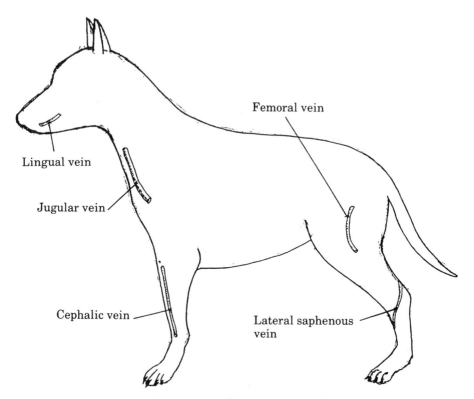

Femoral vein

Lingual vein

Jugular vein

Cephalic vein

Lateral saphenous
vein

Figure 6-7. The position of the major superficial veins.

THE LYMPHATIC SYSTEM

The lymphatic system has a variety of functions in the body, and some of these are relevant to an understanding of the body's fluids (Chapter 5).

Not all the interstitial fluid produced at the capillary bed is resorbed directly into the venous system and the alternative route for drainage of this fluid is provided by the lymphatics. They comprise a network of branching vessels which are present in all tissues of the body, except the brain. The vessels are thin-walled and contain a clear, or slightly white-coloured fluid called lymph. Lymph does not normally contain haemoglobin so in normal tissue the lymphatics are not seen. Flow of lymph occurs in a similar manner to the flow of venous blood, being dependent upon compression by the surrounding muscles aided by valves within the lymphatics which control the direction of flow. Lymph is finally returned to the venous circulation by a small vessel, the thoracic duct, which empties into one of the major veins in the thorax.

Special "filtering stations" called lymph nodes are positioned at strategic points along the lymphatic system. These are sometimes incorrectly called "lymph glands". All lymph has to pass through at least one node before returning to the venous circulation. The lymph nodes destroy or remove

58

abnormal cells or organisms in the lymph. They also produce lymphocytes which play an important role in the immune system of the body, in particular by being responsible for the production of antibodies (immunoglobulins) involved in humoral immunity (Chapter 5).

Lymph nodes are distributed throughout the body (except the brain). Some lie close to the skin and are often palpable in the normal animal (Fig. 6-8). These include:

1. **Submandibular node;** lying at the caudal edge of the angle of mandible, just rostral and lateral to the submandibular salivary gland.

2. **Superficial cervical node;** positioned at the cranial edge of the scapula.

3. **Superficial inguinal node;** lying in the groin.

4. **Popliteal node;** situated at the caudal margin of the stifle joint.

The ease of palpation of the nodes depends both upon their size and on the amount of subcutaneous fat surrounding them. In some animals only the submandibular lymph nodes are palpable.

Lymph nodes will enlarge in response to local disease; for example, an infection in the hindpaw will cause enlargement of the popliteal lymph node.

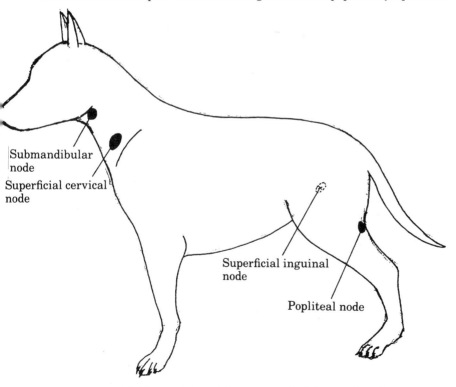

Figure 6-8. The position of the major palpable lymph nodes.

59

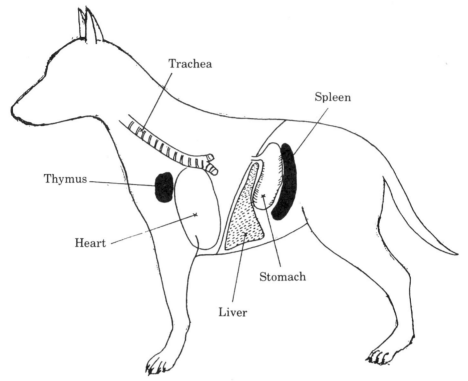

Figure 6-9. Diagram to show the position of the spleen and thymus.

Similarly in cases of neoplasia, tumour cells may spread to the draining lymph nodes where they can establish secondary growths (metastases). A generalised disease process, be it infectious or neoplastic, may cause all lymph nodes to enlarge.

Two important organs are closely related to the lymphatic system; these are the spleen and the thymus. Both have multiple functions, some of which are relevant to the study of body fluids (Chapter 5).

The spleen lies in the abdomen (Fig. 6-9), just caudal to the greater curvature of the stomach. It is a solid organ, normally dark red in colour. It serves multiple functions which include:

1. Production of red blood cells.

2. Destruction of exhausted red blood cells.

3. Production of lymphocytes.

4. Acting as a reservoir of red blood cells: contraction of smooth muscle in the wall of the spleen causes release of red cells into the systemic circulation.

The barbiturate anaesthetic agents (e.g. thiopentone) relax smooth muscle in the spleen, causing a dramatic increase in its size. This explains why the spleen often appears large at laparotomy.

60

The thymus, which lies in the thorax just cranial to the heart, is of greatest importance (and greatest size) in the young animal. It regresses as the animal matures, often disappearing by the time of puberty. The thymus is a further source of lymphocytes and these are closely involved in the mechanisms of cellular immunity. Failure of the thymus to develop in a young animal has a devastating effect on the immune system, leading to an increased susceptibility to disease. On the other hand, the thymus may undergo neoplastic change (as can any of the body's lymphoid tissue) resulting in the condition of thymic lymphosarcoma. This is not uncommon in young cats and causes the thymus to enlarge and press on the surrounding heart, lungs and trachea. In addition, fluid, produced by the tumour, enters the pleural cavity and causes further respiratory embarrassment.

CIRCULATORY FUNCTION: PRESSURE, RESISTANCE AND FLOW

The object of the circulatory system is to provide blood in the arteries at constant pressure, so that the supply to vital tissues, especially the brain and the heart muscle (coronary arteries) never fails. The pressure is generated by the heart and as the blood flows through the major arteries the pressure is maintained. The 'constant' pressure is "mean (average) arterial pressure". The actual pressure varies within each heartbeat, rising to a peak when the ventricles contract and falling to a minimum when they relax. This change of pressure is what you feel when you take the pulse: if it were constant you would feel nothing, whether the pressure was high or low. The fall of pressure during ventricular relaxation (**diastole**) is smoothed out by the elasticity of the major arteries. As the ventricles contract and fill them (**systole**) they expand and during diastole their recoil somewhat reduces the fall in pressure.

The progress from the aorta (the single supply vessel from the left ventricle to all the tissues) to the capillaries is like that from a tree trunk to the finest stems supporting individual leaves. There is progressive subdivision into more and more delicate branches. Between the **arteries** with their combination of elasticity and muscular strength, and the **capillaries** with no more than a single layer of cells to provide the minimum barrier to tissue exchange (Chapter 5) come the muscular **arterioles.** They are a resistance to blood flow and, under control of sympathetic nerves, they can constrict or dilate, increasing or decreasing their resistance. This has great importance in the regulation of arterial pressure and the distribution of blood flow, as we shall see. Functionally, the arterioles provide the **peripheral resistance,** and it is both variable and controllable.

If the arterioles constrict, their resistance increases and this raises the upstream pressure, i.e. it protects the arterial pressure. In fact the interplay between the **cardiac output** (the flow of blood into the aorta) and the **peripheral resistance** which it encounters, both establishes and controls arterial pressure. Constriction of arterioles also drops the downstream pressure – just like standing on a garden hose. It therefore encourages uptake of tissue fluid by reducing **capillary hydrostatic pressure** (Chapter 5). This is useful after a haemorrhage since interstitial fluid is so similar to plasma that its uptake is like internal fluid therapy. The spleen contains a reserve of red cells so that there is the equivalent of an internal blood transfusion. The

61

dominant effect, however, is the uptake of tissue fluid and this causes the haemodilution (fall in PCV) which eventually follows severe or sustained haemorrhage.

The pressure drop across the peripheral resistance is important in protecting the capillaries since they are too flimsy to withstand high pressure. The route from capillaries back to the heart is via the **veins**, at low but measurable pressure. In contrast to arterial pressure, this pressure does not pulsate hence a cut vein bleeds steadily unlike the spurts from a cut artery. Venous pressure rises if the blood fails to pump the returning blood efficiently. The veins are the storage side of the circulatory system; they have muscle (though less than arteries) and can constrict under neural control, thus 'emptying' blood from the storage side to the high pressure side of the system. Again this is a protective aspect of the **'vasoconstriction'** (constriction of blood vessels) which follows haemorrhage. The effects of vasoconstriction are visible because it reduces blood flow to capillaries, hence the pale mucous membranes seen after haemorrhage.

DISTRIBUTION OF BLOOD FLOW

The total volume of the blood vessels far exceeds the available volume of blood – just as the length of a railway network is much greater than the total length of the trains. The effectiveness of both these transport systems depends on correctly distributing the carriers – whether trains or red cells – according to current needs. In particular, the circulatory control centres in the brain have to 'decide' (subconsciously) which tissues are to be generously supplied, because they are active, and which must be temporarily subjected to cuts while they are less active, i.e. which are generously or poorly perfused.

It is impossible to supply all the capillaries at once. Normally they contain only 5% of the available blood but if circulatory regulation failed the entire blood volume could disappear into the capillaries of the liver alone. Thus after a meal the gut is well supplied, muscle and skin less so. In hot surroundings, skin is generously supplied, gut less so. Similarly gut perfusion is restricted during exercise to allow a generous supply to muscle. The combination of a heavy meal and severe exercise, or a heavy meal and a hot bath is dangerous – too much of the circulatory system is demanding supply simultaneously and just like the gas supply before Sunday lunch, there is a danger that pressure cannot be maintained. The combination of fever and exercise is dangerous for similar reasons. Although most tissues 'sacrifice' their perfusion and subsist on less generous blood flow while the other tissues are more active, the brain and the heart muscle are exempt; they always receive the most generous blood supply which is feasible and appropriate.

To a substantial extent tissues also adjust their own blood supply. If they are insufficiently **perfused** (provided with blood) or particularly active, metabolites (end product chemicals from tissue activity) accumulate and relax **precapillary sphincters.** These are bands of muscle which act like taps, opening up access to capillary beds beyond them. Nevertheless the overall control of the circulatory system, and especially the regulation of arterial

62

pressure, depends on the influence of sympathetic nerves on blood vessels, especially arterioles and veins, resetting their patency in response to signals from the circulatory centres of the brain. Any drug which interferes with the effects of sympathetic nerves or the chemical which ultimately produces their effects (noradrenaline, Chapter 10) will impair the regulation of arterial pressure. So may anaesthetics, either by affecting sympathetic nerves or by depressing the circulatory regulation centres of the brain.

DOUBLE CIRCULATION

Though we talk about 'the circulatory system' it is actually a double circulation and the heart is a double pump. The left side provides a high pressure supply of oxygenated blood to the tissues. The right side ensures this supply by receiving the low pressure, low oxygen, venous return and supplying it to the lungs for replenishment (removal of CO_2, replacement of oxygen; Chapter 3).

The blood supply to both the lungs and the remaining tissues needs sufficient pressure to drive it to and through the capillaries. It is the fact that the pulmonary artery contains blood under pressure and therefore has muscular walls which defines it as an artery. The distinction is not based on the chemical composition of the contained blood; the arterial supply to the capillaries of the lungs resembles venous blood in being deoxygenated. Nevertheless the structure of the pulmonary artery is clearly that of an **artery**, i.e. a vessel conducting blood under direct pulse pressure. Similarly the structure of the pulmonary vein clearly identifies it as a **vein,** returning the blood from the lungs to the left side of the heart even though that blood now has the same chemical composition as arterial blood.

You might wonder how the lungs themselves manage, if they receive deoxygenated blood. The answer is that it is the capillaries of the exchange surfaces (alveoli; Chapter 3) which receive blood from the pulmonary artery. The supporting tissues of the lungs are supplied with normal oxygenated arterial blood by the bronchial arteries.

The point of this elaborate double circulation is that the pulmonary capillaries have to be capable of sustaining extremely high blood flow without experiencing high pressure. Excessive pressure would either damage them or cause fluid to flow outwards into the alveolar air cavities (pulmonary oedema; Chapter 5). Then the animal would effectively drown in its own secretions (as it may when pulmonary venous pressure, and therefore capillary pressure, rise as a result of right heart failure or over-rapid administration of intravenous fluids). The solution is to maintain a lower arterial pressure in the pulmonary artery than in the aorta. This works satisfactorily because the lungs do not compete for supply with other tissues, nor do they experience reduced supply (vasoconstriction) during the defence of arterial pressure (which involves the left side of the heart, not the pulmonary artery). Moreover they remain more or less level with or below the heart, regardless of the animal's position, unlike the brain. The lower pressure in the pulmonary artery is reflected by the fact that although its wall is twice as thick as the vena cava, it has only a third of the muscular thickness of the aorta.

REGULATION OF ARTERIAL PRESSURE

The two factors which control arterial pressure, and therefore enable it to be regulated, are cardiac output and peripheral resistance (arteriolar tone or constriction). The greater the cardiac output and the arteriolar resistance, the greater the arterial pressure established by their interaction. The receptors which measure the current value of arterial pressure are placed in the aorta and, appropriately, the carotid arteries, since, of all tissues, the brain is the most susceptible to an inadequate supply pressure (perfusion pressure). Should arterial pressure fall below set point, arterioles are reflexly constricted by sympathetic nerves. Cardiac output is also increased by sympathetic acceleration of heart rate. Both responses are co-ordinated by regulatory centres in the brain.

The greatest problems in stabilising arterial pressure arise from haemorrhage and the main defences are clotting and vasoconstriction (Chapter 5). As already explained, the latter not only protects arterial pressure but draws additional plasma-like fluid back into circulation, from the interstitial fluid. Vasoconstriction is, however, a compromise, a 'tightening of the belt' by less 'important' tissues to allow better pefusion of more vital tissues. The risk is that if the haemorrhage is severe, vasoconstriction may become excessive even in essential organs and damage them; there begins the story of 'circulatory shock' (see below). The first line of defence, however, is invariably to reduce the circulation to skin and visible mucous membranes, hence the pallor which follows haemorrhage. For the same reason, subcutaneously administered fluids are unlikely to be efficiently absorbed in the aftermath of haemorrhage or severe dehydration; there will not be sufficient skin blood flow.

While we have discussed regulation of arterial pressure in relation to the most severe and obvious threat, haemorrhage, the same responses defend against the equally serious depletion of plasma volume which can follow severe dehydration, e.g. associated with diarrhoea (Chapter 8). Clinically, dehydration usually implies the loss of salts, especially sodium, as well as water and since sodium is the osmotic skeleton of ECF (Chapter 5) the result is a loss of plasma but not red cells. The PCV therefore rises, unlike haemorrhage, but the circulating volume falls and undermines the defence of arterial pressure, exactly like haemorrhage.

CARDIAC OUTPUT

The rapid **heart rate** which follows haemorrhage or severe dehydration is already understandable; it is one way of increasing cardiac output in order to maintain arterial pressure. The other is to increase **'stroke volume'**, i.e. the completeness of emptying of the ventricles. The output of a cycle pump can similarly be increased either by pumping faster or by using longer strokes. The sympathetic nerves and the hormone (adrenaline) which has such similar effects, not only accelerate the heart but strengthen its beat. This is one aspect of their general tendency to prepare for 'fright, fight or flight'.

The heart has the very useful property, for a pump, that the more blood it receives (the more it is stretched) the more powerfully it pumps (the stronger

64

the contraction of its muscle). If the heart is routinely accustomed to hard work it also thickens its muscle and thus enlarges; the hearts of athletes 'hypertrophy' just like the muscles of their legs or arms.

All adaptations have their limits. The failing heart is also enlarged (and rounded, as seen on x-ray), but this is a flabby heart overstretched by its inability to efficiently eject the blood which it receives. This might result from inherent weakness of the muscle, or damage, or from leakage within the heart (see below). Acceleration of heart rate has its limits; the heart needs a reasonable period of relaxation (diastole) in order to fill and to receive its own blood supply. During contraction (systole) blood flow to its own muscle is restricted by compression. Very high heart rates therefore prevent the heart muscle from being properly oxygenated and the ventricles from filling sufficiently to sustain maximum cardiac output.

PULSE AND HEART SOUNDS: VENTRICULAR FUNCTION AND FAILURE

Both the pulse and the heart sounds tell us mainly about ventricular function. In fact the pulse reflects the output of the left ventricle since the output of the right ventricle is received exclusively by the lungs. The fullness of the pulse depends on the ability of the left ventricle to raise systolic pressure above diastolic, and upon the resistance offered by the arterioles. The pulse rate directly indicates heart rate unless the ventricles contract when they are too poorly filled to produce a beat in the pulse; a heart beat is still audible in the chest. By listening with the stethoscope (auscultation) and comparing with the pulse we feel (palpate) we may thus detect a 'pulse deficit'. The regularity and rate of the pulse otherwise reflect the rate and regularity of ventricular acitivity, since both ventricles contract together. The main reasons for an elevated heart rate are fever or sympathetic activity, the latter associated with fear, activity or compensation for either inadequate cardiac output (reduced circulating volume or heart failure) or reduced haemoglobin concentration (anaemia; Chapter 3).

As the ventricles contract their entry valves close (**atrio-ventricular or A-V valves**). This causes the **first heart sound** ('lub'). During contraction the exit valves are open but when systole is complete and the ventricles begin to relax, their pressure begins to fall below aortic pressure. Their exit valves (aortic and pulmonic) therefore close and produce the **second heart sound** ('dup'). The first sound is longer and lower (in pitch and position of clearest sound) than the second. At resting heart rates the interval between first and second (systole) is shorter than that between second and the first sound of the next beat.

Normal heart sounds are not actually caused by 'slamming' of the valves but by the turbulent blood flow associated with closure. If the closed valves fail to fulfill their function, i.e. to provide a watertight seal, leakage of blood will cause additional turbulence and additional abnormal heart sounds called **'murmurs'**. A leaking entry valve will therefore cause a murmur during systole, by allowing blood to squirt back into the atria instead of all being propelled into the aorta or pulmonary artery. Very reasonably, such a valve is

65

described as 'incompetent'. A leaking exit valve allows blood to re-enter the ventricles during diastole instead of remaining within the aorta or pulmonary artery. In both cases, the heart inefficiently 'recycles' some of the blood instead of propelling it towards the tissues; cardiac output is therefore reduced and there is some degree of heart failure.

Narrowing of the valves (**stenosis**) can also cause both turbulence (murmurs) and an obstruction to blood flow (therefore heart failure). This time the defective A-V valve, if stenotic, is heard to murmur at diastole because blood flows through the narrowed opening during ventricular filling. Similarly, the stenotic exit valve (aortic or pulmonic) is heard to murmur at systole because it impedes the emptying of the ventricles into the aorta and pulmonary artery.

Other vascular abnormalities may cause audible turbulence and murmurs, e.g. defective partitioning between the left and right side of the heart or persistence of the foetal by-pass vessel (ductus arteriosus) which allows blood to short-circuit the lungs during pregnancy (when the placenta oxygenates foetal blood). Blood is "thicker than water" and its greater viscosity makes it more resistant to turbulence. Anaemia or haemodilution may, however, reduce viscosity sufficiently to allow turbulence and murmurs even within a normal heart. Any murmur is likely to be more audible after exercise, when cardiac output is increased, flow rates are higher and turbulence is therefore more probable.

Incompetent valves can obviously cause heart failure by allowing back-leakage of blood. They can also result from heart failure, however, because a weak and failing heart becomes overexpanded (dilated) and its valves may no longer seal properly. Whatever the cause of heart failure it can initially affect either the left or right side alone. Since one of the main effects of heart failure is to cause oedema (Chapter 5) this can affect most tissues except the lungs in the case of right-sided heart failure (raised pressure in the venous system and, therefore, the capillaries). More seriously, in the case of left-sided heart failure, pressure rises in the pulmonary veins and causes pulmonary oedema. By the time heart failure is advanced it usually involves both sides (i.e. it is 'bilateral').

You will notice that our discussion of heart function and heart failure has centred on the ventricles and almost ignored the atria. This is perfectly reasonable since they do little more than boost ventricular filling. At rest, this contribution is quite unimportant and surprising degress of exertion can be achieved with totally disrupted atrial function, as in atrial fibrillation. Indeed the main danger of this condition is not from the defective atrial function but the potential effect on ventricular activity. Which brings us to the co-ordination of heart function.

CO-ORDINATION OF HEART FUNCTION: DYSRHYTHMIAS

You have probably heard the results of incoordinate heart function through a stethoscope or felt it as an irregular pulse. These **dysrhythmias** (disturbances of rhythm) are important because they can both disrupt heart function and result from cardiac failure (through cardiac enlargement or damage). The question is why is the rhythm of the normal heart so steady?

The answer is that rhythm is built into heart muscle even in the early embryo when there is scarcely a heart at all. The key to a normal cardiac rhythm is that all chambers are paced by a single dominant pacemaker (the **sinoatrial** or **'S-A' node**, in the right atrium). In order to maintain dominance, its natural frequency is faster than the natural frequency of the atria or ventricles. Pacing is achieved by rhythmic changes of voltage (just as with an artificial pacemaker). The electrical activity spreads swiftly through the atria and triggers their muscle to contract. At the junction with the ventricles (A-V node) it is delayed, allowing time for completion of ventricular filling. Then the electrical acitivity spreads through the ventricles along special fast-conduction pathways which ensure rapid and organised transmission. The result is to trigger a fast, powerful ventricular contraction in the appropriate pattern to achieve efficient emptying.

Sometimes odd beats fall to produce electrical activity beyond the A-V node; the atria contract but because the ventricles do not, there is neither a pulse wave nor *any* heart sound (remember, the ventricles 'drive' *both* heart sounds). This is a 'dropped beat'. Sometimes, in disease, animals have atrial fibrillation. This means that there is no co-ordinated atrial activity. Instead, the electrical activity and the contractions are rather random and accordingly the A-V node is activated irregularly – sometimes too fast to respond to every activation. The result is a chaotic ventricular rhythm. The ventricles still supply a substantial cardiac output but less efficiently because of their irregular rhythm. The main danger, however, is that the ventricles themselves may be thrown into fibrillation, i.e. incoordinate, ineffective contractions. There is then little if any cardiac output, i.e. there is sudden death.

Complete heart block sounds a very alarming condition but need not be so. It means that no electrical activity passes from the atria to the ventricles via the A-V node. The ventricles, therefore, unlike the atria, can no longer be driven by the rhythm of the pacemaker. Instead they reveal their own slower natural rhythm, i.e. they beat at a different frequency to the atria. It may be inefficient and it indicates underlying disease but it is far from lethal.

When the heart is performing with normal rhythm, responding to the natural pacemaker of the S-A node it is said to be in 'sinus rhythm'. Normal dogs often show an irregularity of rhythm which is perfectly harmless and is caused by a fluctuating frequency of the pacemaker. It is therefore called 'sinus arrhythmia'. It results from changes in neural activity and thoracic blood flow associated with breathing; these accelerate heart rate during inspiration.

You may have seen electrocardiograms, ECG's. These are records of the electrical activity of the heart, obtained from leads applied to the animal's limbs (usually). If you have seen them look at Fig. 6-10, for interest, but if you have not, do not worry. The electrical activity (depolarisation) triggering the atria generates the 'P' wave of the ECG. The activity triggering the ventricles causes the QRS complex and the gap between them reflects the delay in

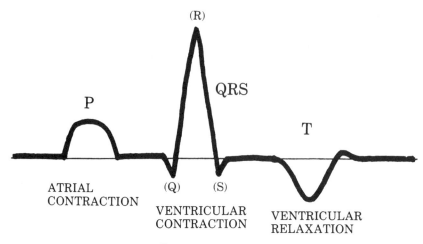

Figure 6-10. E.C.G.

conduction at the A-V node. The T wave is caused by the electrical 'resetting' (repolarisation) of the ventricles. The shape, size and relationships between these waves can reveal or confirm a great deal about disturbances of cardiac rhythm and their implications for the animal's future health.

CIRCULATORY SHOCK

One of the most interesting illustrations of the interaction between physiology and disease is the condition known as 'shock'. There are several causes and more than one type but the essential features are shared and best illustrated by 'traumatic', 'hypovolaemic' or 'haemorrhagic' shock, i.e. shock due to injury, severe dehydration or haemorrhage.

The initial response to a loss of circulating volume, as we have seen, is vasoconstriction. It is protective because it supports arterial pressure and allows replenishment of plasma volume from tissue fluid. The response tends to correct the disturbance; negative feedback (Chapter 1 and Fig. 6-11). But if it lasts too long, and is too widespread, capillaries may become damaged and, therefore, leaky (Chapter 5). Now we have additional fluid loss and a response which amplifies the disturbance, i.e. positive feedback (Chapter 1 and Fig. 6-11). As shock progresses, more such vicious circles are established. The loss of plasma from capillaries leaves behind blood with a very high PCV (red cell content). It is, therefore, very viscous, sticky, difficult to circulate through capillaries. Since good perfusion depends not just on the **presence** of blood in capillaries but its efficient **flow** through them, capillary perfusion deteriorates and the likelihood of damage to both capillaries and tissues increases (Fig. 6-11).

Eventually, because of the metabolites accumulating from poorly perfused tissues, the precapillary sphincters relax. This intensifies the problems because the diminished volume of blood now has access to an increased volume of vessels; it may become impossible to maintain arterial pressure.

68

Yet capillary pressure tends to rise (Fig. 6-11) encouraging fluid to leave the capillaries rather than re-enter them and intensifying the fall in circulating volume which started the whole sad cycle of events.

Shock is therefore, a progressive sequence of vicious circles, each leading to the next. It is a caricature of the physiological response to haemorrhage. The features are still recognisable but they have become exaggerated to an absurd and damaging degree. The solution is to replace circulating volume and to do so urgently, before the vicious circles progress too far. The amounts of fluid needed may be large, because the damaged capillaries make the circulatory system 'leaky'. Unless the PCV is extremely low the replacement fluids need not include blood because, by reducing viscosity, a slight fall in PCV actually improves blood flow and oxygen delivery. A high PCV may make it virtually impossible for blood to flow efficiently through capillaries.

Whatever is done needs to be done fast because the condition is so progressive. Soldiers wounded in the Vietnam War were much more effectively treated for shock than those in earlier wars. The key factor was not the arrival of new drugs but the arrival of rescue helicopters to allow established drugs (especially intravenous fluids) to be used sooner. Other than further fluid loss, delay is the biggest enemy in treating shock.

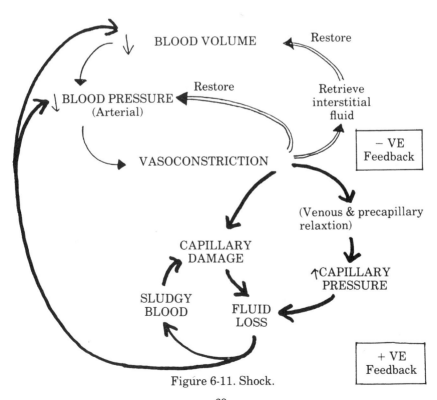

Figure 6-11. Shock.

69

CHAPTER 7:
URINARY SYSTEM

THIRST AND DEHYDRATION

It may seem strange to begin a consideration of the urinary system with thirst, but without it the urinary system would have little opportunity to function.

Animals and people lose water continuously – to different extents and by different routes but unavoidably. The water losses in urine and faeces are controllable but those through skin (even without sweating) and the humidification of respired air are not. Lactation imposes an additional need for water and so, to a lesser extent, does pregnancy. The need to drink is, therefore, an even more constant feature of mammalian life than the need to eat and the maintenance of a constant body water (Chapter 5) depends on both thirst and renal function. Humans, because they drink tasty liquids, tend to consume excess and excrete the surplus (especially with some liquids!). In contrast, dogs when they drink water tend to drink according to need and so maintain a relatively constant output of concentrated urine. With flavoured drinks (milk, soups, etc.) they behave more like people. Cats can produce even higher concentrations of urine than dogs.

Three signals trigger drinking. In decreasing order of importance they are:

1. Increased osmotic concentration of body fluids (detected by 'osmoreceptors' in the hypothalamus of the brain): too many salty crisps, too much water loss.
2. Reduced volume of ECF and especially plasma: the reason that casualties often crave water, despite their more serious problems.
3. Dry mouth: talking too much in a hot, dry room.

In addition to these signals of a need for water some drinking is a matter of established habit at particular times of day. Need-driven drinking has a threshold, which is fortunate or we would be sipping non-stop to replace the continuous losses through the skin and during breathing. Nevertheless drinking is a sensitive regulator of the osmotic concentration of body fluids and will be triggered by an increase of less than 1%. In a 20 kg dog the water intake required to correct a 1% increase in osmolarity (osmotic concentration) will be around 120 ml – about a wine-glass.

Drinking is not the only source of water; the food also contains water and animals on dry diets will drink far more than those on moister food. A small amount of water is also generated by the chemical reactions of metabolism. Although animals may occasionally develop overdrinking as a form of abnormal behaviour, drinking is mostly highly attuned to need and the usual reason for an increase ('polydipsia') is genuine dehydration. Water intake must never, therefore, be restricted without a first class clinical reason and even then, only with careful surveillance of bodyweight.

Dehydration can deplete an animal of 5% of its bodyweight with little visible effect yet by the time the losses progress to 15% of bodyweight the effects are likely to be severe and potentially lethal. Clinically important fluid deficits (requiring replacement by fluid therapy) are therefore likely to fall in the range 50-200 ml/kg bodyweight. The seriousness of a particular level of dehydration will depend on the accompanying salt loss. Since sodium provides the osmotic skeleton of ECF (Chapter 5), the greater the sodium deficit the greater the reduction in ECF volume, including plasma, and the greater the risk of circulatory collapse (Chapter 6).

RENAL FUNCTION: GENERAL

Renal function has some rather curious features. The most obvious function of the kidney is to produce urine – yet strangely, the most common sign of failing kidneys is that they produce **too much** urine. This reminds us that the essential role of the kidneys is to restrict water loss, ideally producing the smallest amount of urine needed to excrete the end-products of nitrogen (protein) metabolism and excess dietary salts. The end-products of carbohydrate and fat metabolism (CO_2 and water) do not rely on renal excretion. The kidneys are also important for the excretion of some poisons (including drugs) though they may be damaged in the process.

The two kidneys receive up to a quarter of the cardiac output – far more than the brain, yet even a single kidney is more than sufficient to sustain normal life. Of the plasma received, about 20% is converted to primitive urine and then the kidney spends most of its considerable oxygen and energy consumption retrieving about 99% of this primitive urine. Just as well: each day's primitive urine is equivalent to about 4 months' final urine output. One hour's primitive urine, if excreted, would produce severe dehydration (15% bodyweight).

In fact the main function of the kidney is to regulate the volume and composition of the extracellular fluid. It is also an endocrine organ, i.e. one which produces hormones (Chapter 9). These include:

(a) **Erythropoietin** which allows the maturation of red cells (hence one reason for anaemia in chronic renal failure, CRF).

(b) The most active form of **vitamin D** which allows adequate intestinal calcium absorption (hence one reason for bone damage in CRF).

72

(c) **Renin** which in turn generates **angiotensin** in circulation: this affects thirst, arterial pressure and sodium excretion (one reason for high blood pressure with renal disease, though not the usual one – and much less often in dogs than in people). The kidney also breaks down some hormones, hence CRF, among its many effects, can cause endocrine disturbances.

SODIUM AND WATER

Since sodium is the osmotic skeleton of ECF, the balance between dietary sodium intake and renal sodium retention controls the volume of the ECF. The concentration of the retained sodium is regulated by increases or decreases in body water, i.e. by thirst and renal water retention. The latter is controlled by the hormone ADH (**antidiuretic hormone**). Despite being called a posterior pituitary hormone, ADH is produced in the adjacent hypothalamus. The posterior pituitary simply acts as a store. The stimuli which release ADH are exactly like the two main stimuli for thirst; an increase in the osmotic concentration of ECF (and thus of ICF too) or a loss of ECF volume, especially circulating volume. Though both thirst and ADH primarily defend plasma sodium concentration, severe depletion of plasma volume becomes an overriding reason for water retention. Thirst and ADH will then depress plasma sodium concentration instead of regulating it; the attempt to boost ECF volume takes priority. This is the usual reason for a fall of plasma sodium concentration and it explains why correction does not require high-sodium fluids, merely restoration of plasma volume (with solutions of plasma-like sodium concentration).

The beauty of the dual-control of body water is illustrated by the unusual but interesting condition of diabetes insipidus, defective production or effectiveness of ADH. (Diabetes mellitus, sugar diabetes, is different – excessive blood sugar, usually a lack of the pancreatic hormone insulin, Chapter 8). Since the kidney cannot conserve water properly without ADH you would expect diabetes insipidus to elevate plasma sodium concentration. But this triggers thirst and the end result is not a rise of plasma sodium but a compensatory (and massive) polydipsia.

NEPHRON FUNCTION: GLOMERULAR FILTRATION

Each kidney consists of thousands of nephrons which, for all practical purposes, function identically. A nephron begins with a blind sac (Bowman's capsule) into which is thrust a capillary tuft (the glomerulus) like a fist into a very soft balloon (Fig. 7-2). The process of **glomerular filtration** involves the pressure-driven transfer of water and solutes from plasma, through the glomerular membrane, into Bowman's space, the true beginning of the urinary tract. From here each nephron consists of a **proximal tubule**, still within the outer part of the kidney, the **cortex** (Fig. 7-1, 7-2). Then the nephron dips deep into the inner part of the kidney (the **medulla**) before doubling back like a hairpin and thus forming the '**loop of Henle**'. The nephron returns to the cortex (distal tubule) before diving back through the medulla and joining with adjacent nephrons in the **collecting ducts** which ultimately empty, via the 'renal pelvis' into the ureters. The **ureters** conduct

1) Complete

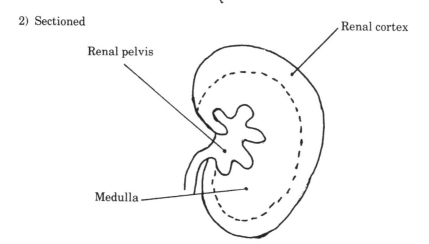

Hilus

Renal artery

Renal vein

Ureter

2) Sectioned

Renal cortex

Renal pelvis

Medulla

Figure 7-1. Structure of the kidney.

urine from the kidneys to the bladder, not by gravity but by co-ordinated squeezing contractions ('peristalsis', as in the intestine, Chapter 8).

These 'to-ings' and 'fro-ings' have a sensible functional explanation as we shall see in the next section. Meanwhile it is important to emphasise that the glomerulus acts as a filter, restraining molecules the size of the main plasma protein (albumin) or larger. It also restrains substances bound to these proteins – for example many hormones and much of the calcium in plasma. Anything smaller and freely dissolved (sugars, amino acids, salts, smaller proteins) appears in primitive urine.

The fact that small proteins can enter urine is illustrated by the fact that both myoglobin and haemoglobin can appear in urine if they are released into plasma by muscle damage or red cell damage, respectively. In normal

74

animals, the amount of protein in primitive urine is small and much is reabsorbed in the proximal tubule. The main reasons, therefore, for the appearance of large amounts of protein in the urine are:

(a) Addition of blood or inflammatory exudates from a damaged bladder
(b) Leakage of protein through damaged glomeruli.

Renal disease does not invariably cause sufficient glomerular damage to produce proteinuria.

Glomerular filtration is the foundation of renal function and its decline is the hallmark of renal failure. The high rate of glomerular filtration is heavily dependent on adequate renal perfusion (which can be undermined by anaesthesia). Normally the kidney is 'spared' during vasoconstriction in response to haemorrhage and the glomeruli are able to maintain their perfusion pressure despite falls in arterial pressure, but there is a limit to this.

TUBULAR FUNCTION: PROXIMAL TUBULE

The proximal tubule allows additional substances to enter urine by secretion. This is important because it may include solutes unable to cross the

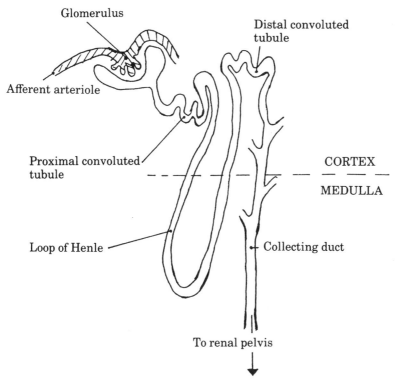

Figure 7-2. Diagram to show the structure of the nephron.

75

glomerular barrier and it can also allow substances to enter primitive urine at a concentration higher than plasma (unlike glomerular filtration). Many drugs and toxins are excreted in this way, some after preliminary processing by the liver. Because it experiences high concentrations, the proximal tubule may be damaged in the process of excreting poisons. A certain amount of cell damage, fortunately, is reversible. The proximal tubule (like the distal tubule) is also important in excreting hydrogen ions (H^+) into urine.

The main function of the proximal tubule is to reabsorb about two-thirds of the primitive urine, along with the useful substances in it. Thus primitive urine contains the same glucose concentration as plasma but healthy final urine contains none; the proximal tubule reabsorbs it all. It has, however, a maximum speed of reabsorption for many substances including glucose. Thus, if blood glucose reaches a certain level, primitive urine contains too much to allow complete reabsorption and glucose appears in final urine – this is the explanation for the 'glycosuria' of diabetes mellitus; it warns us of an elevated blood sugar.

The proximal tubule achieves its reabsorption by retrieving sodium and uses a lot of energy to do so. Water follows, osmotically, and the concentration of other solutes rises, encouraging their own reabsorption. The exception is the nitrogenous waste products (urea, creatinine); they remain in the primitive urine and become more concentrated as its volume shrinks.

Since the fluid reabsorbed in the proximal tubule is exactly like glomerular filtrate and thus resembles plasma, but without the nitrogenous waste, it is an ideal ECF. Appropriately the amount of reabsorption increases when plasma volume needs to be restored and it falls when plasma volume is excessive. Inevitably the delivery of urine to the rest of the nephron will also be affected, sometimes with adverse effects, as we shall see.

LOOP

If plasma is too concentrated we need to retain water to dilute it; we therefore need to concentrate the urine, i.e. to retrieve more water from it. Similarly if plasma is diluted by too much water the remedy is to excrete more water, i.e. to produce a dilute urine. The loop is the basis of both concentration and dilution of urine. Essentially, the ascending limb extracts salt with very little water into the interstitial fluid of the medulla which therefore becomes very concentrated (Fig. 7-3). At the same time the urine becomes very dilute and, if left unchanged, will remove large amounts of water from the body; this is the dilute urine which underlies diabetes insipidus. Additional dilution occurs in the distal tubule when sodium is conserved.

On the other hand, when water needs to be conserved, the concentrated medullary interstitial fluid created by the loop provides the means of doing so. If the collecting ducts become leaky, rather than impermeable, osmosis will extract water from the urine which they contain and make it concentrated. This is how ADH acts; it relies on the osmotic gradient provided by the concentrated interstitial fluid surrounding the collecting ducts in the medulla. Concentrated urine has both a high specific gravity and a high osmolarity – the latter is the more accurate measure of its high osmotic concentration.

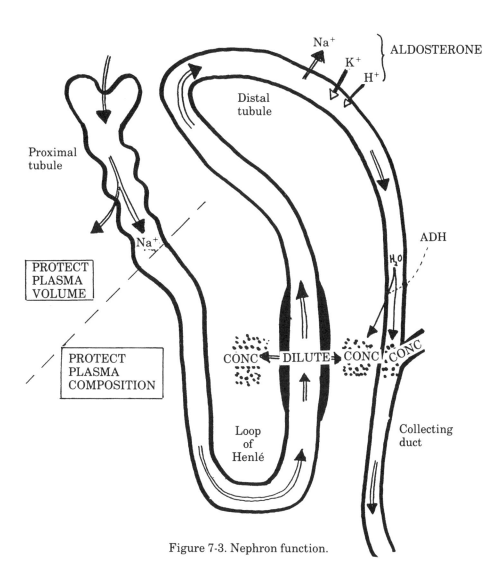

Figure 7-3. Nephron function.

Interestingly, two conditions keep the collecting duct impermeable and therefore cause polyuria (excess urine output) which, in turn, causes a compensatory polydipsia. One is Cushing's syndrome (production of excess adrenal corticosteroids) and the other is a raised blood calcium (hypercalcaemia – sometimes caused by a tumour). The most common cause of polyuria, however, is damage to the renal medulla and hence to the renal concentrating mechanism as in chronic renal failure. The deterioration of plasma composition may also contribute by making the kidney less able to respond to ADH.

DISTAL TUBULE

Though most sodium is reabsorbed in the proximal tubule (two-thirds) and loop (one-quarter), the remaining reabsorption in the distal tubule has special importance. First, it sets the final urinary loss of sodium which, in the long term, must balance the dietary intake. Second, when the animal is 'volume depleted' and desperately needs to retain sodium in order to boost ECF volume, urine (like faeces) can become virtually free of sodium. Urinary and faecal sodium conservation are regulated by a hormone, **aldosterone**, from the adrenal cortex.

Aldosterone production is linked to ECF volume by the kidney itself; when ECF volume falls the supply arterioles of the glomeruli respond to their declining perfusion by liberating renin. This generates angiotensin in the plasma which, in turn, stimulates the adrenals to release aldosterone. The negative feedback loop is complete (Fig. 7-4). Sodium conservation in the distal tubule (and large intestine) also helps the excretion of potassium, by an indirect exchange. Appropriately, a rise in plasma potassium directly stimulates aldosterone secretion, thus helping to correct the rise by increasing potassium excretion (Fig. 7-4). It also helps to drive potassium into

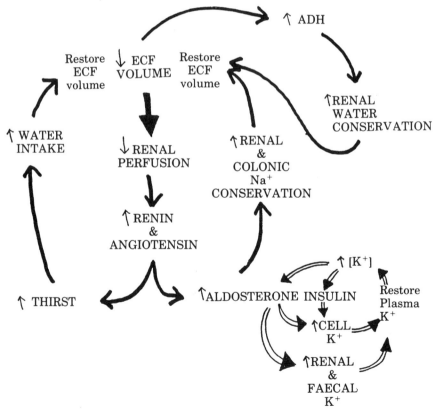

Figure 7-4. Regulation of ECF volume and K^+

78

cells, as does insulin, further protecting plasma potassium from elevation (Chapter 5). The distal tubule also helps the regulation of acid-base balance by acidifying urine, i.e. secreting hydrogen ions (see below).

The regulation of water balance (therefore plasma sodium), plasma potassium and pH (hydrogen ion concentration) all depend on processes beyond the proximal tubule. Excessive reabsorption of fluid in the proximal tubule can thus restrict delivery to the sites responsible for these regulatory functions and undermine their effectiveness. The main cause of enhanced or excessive reabsorption in the proximal tubule is a depleted ECF volume. Repair of ECF volume, with plasma-like electrolyte solutions, thus improves not only its volume but also its composition by restoring the regulatory ability of the kidney. This, together with the prevention of shock, makes repair of ECF volume the paramount objective of fluid therapy. Obviously it can only be achieved with solutions containing plasma-like concentrations of sodium (130-150 mmol/l).

ACID-BASE BALANCE

We have already encountered the fact that the kidneys act alongside the liver in metabolising and excreting drugs and poisons. They also act together with the liver and the lungs to regulate acid-base balance, i.e. to stabilise plasma H^+ concentration (normally measured as pH).
The key to a stable plasma pH is the action of buffer solutions which yield H^+ to bolster a falling hydrogen ion concentration (rising pH) or combine with H^+ to prevent a rise in plasma hydrogen ion concentration (fall in pH). The two most important buffers in blood are haemoglobin and, above all, bicarbonate (throughout ECF).

$$HHb \rightleftharpoons H^+ + Hb^- \qquad (a)$$
$$\text{Haemoglobin}$$

$$H_2O + CO_2 \longleftrightarrow H_2CO_3 \rightleftharpoons H^+ + HCO_3- \qquad (b)$$
$$\text{Bicarbonate}$$

(The dotted half-arrows combat alkalinisation, the solid
half-arrows combat acidification.)

The true cause of acidity is the free hydrogen ion concentration (H^+) and the simplest way of removing hydrogen ions is to combine them with buffer anions (negative ions) such as haemoglobin or bicarbonate.

From equation (b) we can see that effectively

$$H^+ \quad \alpha \quad \frac{CO_2}{HCO_3^-}$$

i.e. that hydrogen ion concentration depends on the ratio of concentration of CO_2 and bicarbonate. If the ratio is normal, so is the plasma H^+ and pH. The special importance of the bicarbonate buffer system is therefore that its components, CO_2 and bicarbonate, can be controlled, the former by pulmonary ventilation and the latter by renal bicarbonate reabsorption.

Since bicarbonate is the main buffer of ECF it is important that solutions for repair of ECF volume contain plasma-like amounts of bicarbonate, to avoid diluting it. Often they contain lactate because healthy liver has a great capacity to convert lactate to bicarbonate, as necessary (e.g. after vigorous sprinting). Brief periods of anaerobic metabolism (Chapter 3) generate lactic acid and thus consume bicarbonate buffer; when the oxygen supply is restored the lactate is metabolised and bicarbonate is regenerated. (The preference for lactate over bicarbonate is largely a matter of manufacturers' convenience and, slightly, protection against overdose since the conversion to bicarbonate is gradual.)

Buffers are also important in urine because, by taking up H^+, they increase the amount of H^+ which can be carried by urine at a given pH (i.e. much more H^+ is carried tied to buffers than free in solution). The main urinary buffer is phosphate (from plasma). Without urine buffers even the most strongly acid urine (pH 4.5) could only eliminate the H^+ in 60 ml of gastric fluid by using one ton to do it! This 'transport' function of buffers is also important in plasma, allowing H^+ to be harmlessly transported from sites of production, e.g. active liver or muscle, to the site of excretion, the kidney, without disturbing plasma pH.

RENAL DISEASE

We already remarked that one kidney is more than enough to sustain life. In fact the greater the loss of nephrons, e.g. through disease, the harder the surviving nephrons work to compensate (i.e. their individual turnover of filtration and reabsorption increases to limit the overall fall in glomerular filtration). Animals may therefore look healthy with two-thirds of their renal function lost. They are, however, much less adaptable to everyday events such as changes in diet, heat stress, dehydration, diarrhoea, because so much of the kidney's compensatory range is already engaged in simply keeping the animal stable. Additional stresses are no longer within the range for which the kidney can compensate.

The clinical problems encountered are easily predicted from the range of renal functions and disturbances already discussed; e.g. bone damage, anaemia, polyuria and polydipsia, abnormalities of plasma H^+ and K^+. In addition, since nitrogenous waste products such as urea and creatinine rely on the kidney for excretion, their plasma concentration rises in CRF. They are not themselves, particularly toxic (you would not want a major excretory product to be toxic!) but they warn us of other accumulating nitrogenous waste products that contribute to the characteristic biochemical illness of advanced CRF; 'uraemia'. Part of the treatment of CRF is to reduce protein intake in an attempt to control blood urea. It is important to realise, however, that the associated fall in blood urea does not indicate improved renal function. It merely indicates that with less protein consumed, the liver produces less urea. More important, the body produces less of the toxic end-products of protein metabolism which the kidneys can no longer excrete.

DIURETICS

These drugs are used to increase urine output and, notably, sodium excretion. The reason for the latter proviso is that the main clinical use is to get rid of

80

oedema, i.e. excess interstitial fluid (Chapter 5). Since this is ECF, the aim is clearly to reduce excess ECF volume and the way to do this is to reduce its osmotic skeleton, i.e. to reduce body sodium.

Sometimes the kidneys themselves cause oedema by allowing excessive protein leakage through damaged glomeruli (Chapter 5). Even where the primary cause lies elsewhere, e.g. failure of the liver to produce enough albumin or a raised venous pressure due to cardiac failure (Chapter 5, 6) the kidneys remain substantially responsible. The reason is that oedema involves the expansion of the major component of ECF (interstitial fluid) from the minor component (plasma). It could not continue unless the kidneys, as they invariably do, maintain their commitment to restore plasma volume. Thus the kidneys are always the 'enabling' cause of oedema even when they are not the main cause. It is therefore, perhaps, less surprising that diuretics, which act mainly on the kidney, may be used to treat various forms of oedema which, at first sight, seem to have little to do with renal function.

BLADDER: MICTURITION

The bladder stores urine inertly, without altering its composition, until the tension in its walls triggers the complex spinal reflex, micturition, which empties the bladder into the urethra. At the same time the contracting bladder muscle (detrusor) seals the ureters and prevents backflow of urine. During urine storage the bladder expands without exerting pressure on its contents, and thus without opposing the addition of urine from the ureters. Although micturition is basically a sacral spinal reflex (Chapter 10) both complete emptying and voluntary control (housetraining) require the intact influence of higher centres, notably in the brain. Hence bladder function is easily disrupted by spinal injury. The main risk of disrupted bladder function, apart from pain, is infection with the risk of it spreading back to the kidneys.

ANATOMY OF THE URINARY SYSTEM

Having studied in some detail the mutliple functions of the urinary system, and, in particular, the kidneys, it is necessary to consider the anatomy of this region. It can be divided into two sections:

1. **Upper urinary tract;** comprises the kidneys, ureters and bladder. The anatomy of this area differs little between males and females.

2. **Lower urinary tract;** comprises the urethra and associated structures. There are major anatomical differences in this region between males and females.

THE UPPER URINARY TRACT

The kidneys are paired structures lying dorsally in the abdominal cavity, one on either side of the vertebral column. The right kidney lies slightly more cranial than the left. The kidneys are protected by the overlying sublumbar muscles and by the lumbar vertebrae. In the dog, it is unusual to feel either kidney when palpating the abdomen, whereas in the cat the kidneys are easily palpated and are quite mobile within the abdomen, especially the left.

81

Kidneys are normally dark red/brown in colour, and are covered by a thick fibrous capsule which is white. If a kidney is cut open to reveal the internal architecture (Fig. 7-1), two main areas are visible:

1. **The Renal Cortex**
   This is superficial (closer to the outer surface) and contains the glomerulus, and the proximal and distal tubules of the nephrons.

2. **The Renal Medulla**
   This lies deep to the cortex, and contains the loop of Henle of the nephrons as well as the collecting ducts (Fig. 7-2).

Blood is supplied to the kidney by the renal artery (normally one artery per kidney), and blood is drained by the renal vein (again, one per kidney). Both the renal artery and vein are relatively large vessels – this is not unexpected when one considers the high blood flow to the kidneys. Having entered the kidney the renal artery divides and gives off a large number of branches which spread out through the substance of the kidney and give rise to the afferent arterioles which supply the glomeruli. Each glomerulus, unusually, is drained by another arteriole (efferent) instead of a vein: this allows the contraction of these two types of arteriole to stabilise the pressure within the glomerulus even if arterial pressure changes.

Urine produced by the nephrons flows along a series of collecting ducts to an area called the renal pelvis. This is situated deep in the medulla, close to the area where the blood vessels enter and leave the kidney. Urine next flows from the renal pelvis into the ureter. This is a thin tube which passes caudally from the kidney to the bladder. The wall of the ureter is composed of fibrous tissue and smooth muscle which propels urine along the ureter by peristalsis, normally only in one direction (from the kidney to the bladder).

The bladder is the main storage organ for urine. It lies on the floor of the pelvis and normally extends cranially into the abdomen. The wall of the bladder contains smooth (non-striated) muscle, and the thickness of the wall varies according to the amount of urine stored in the bladder. As urine accumulates in the bladder it expands, extending both cranially and dorsally, into the abdominal cavity.

The two ureters enter the bladder dorsally (at an area called the trigone) and they pass through the bladder wall at an acute angle; this creates a valve mechanism which normally prevents urine passing from the bladder back up the ureters.

Urine leaves the bladder via the urethra which is part of the lower urinary tract.

THE LOWER URINARY TRACT

In both the male and female the urethra is a fibromuscular tube which allows urine to pass out from the bladder at the time of micturition. However, when urine is being stored in the bladder the urethra acts as a valve (by virtue of the

82

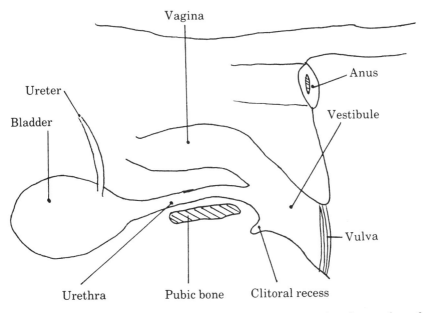

CRANIAL   CAUDAL

Vagina

Anus

Ureter

Vestibule

Bladder

Vulva

Urethra   Pubic bone   Clitoral recess

Figure 7-5. Longitudinal section of the pelvis, demonstrating the urethra of the bitch.

muscle in its wall) and prevents flow of urine, thereby maintaining continence. There are major differences between the male and female in this section of the urinary tract, so each is now considered separately.

The Female

The urethra is relatively short compared with the male. It runs caudally from the bladder on the floor of the pelvis to enter the vestibule. The latter is a short muscular tube which continues caudoventrally and terminates at the vulva; it serves as the common opening for both the urinary and genital systems (Fig. 7-5).

Catheterisation of the bladder in the bitch (or queen) requires a sound knowledge of the local regional anatomy. It is necessary to locate the opening of the urethra on the floor of the vestibule; this is most easily achieved by positioning the animal on its back and introducing a speculum to temporarily dilate the vulva and vestibule. Just inside the vulva, on the floor of the vestibule is the clitoris, and lying on either side are two small blind-ending recesses. These should not be mistaken for the urethral opening which is situated more cranially (and is not a paired structure). The urethral orifice normally offers little resistance to the passage of a catheter; in contrast the clitoral recesses are blind-ending and will not permit the passage of a catheter.

83

The Male

In the male, the urethra is part of both the urinary and genital systems, serving to transport urine from the bladder, and semen (sperm plus seminal fluids) to the vagina (at the time of mating).

In comparison with the female the male's urethra is much longer, especially in the dog. In the latter, the urethra commences at the bladder and runs caudally on the floor of the pelvis, ventral to the rectum. It passes through the prostate gland, and in this region the two deferent ducts (coming from the testes) join the urethra. The urethra continues caudally to reach the ischial arch where it bends ventrally through approximately 160 degrees (nearly a half-circle). The urethra next passes into the penis, running ventral to the os penis (the bone within the penis), and finally opens at the external urethral orifice (located at the tip of the penis) (Fig. 7-6). The penis itself is protected by

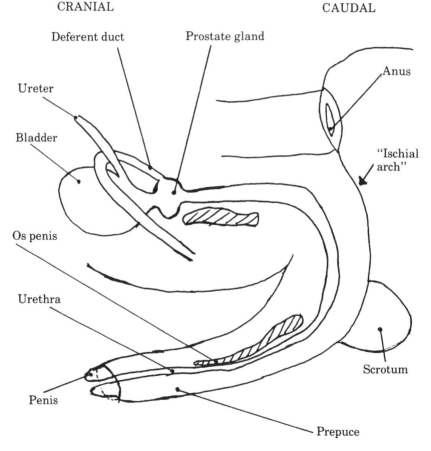

CRANIAL   CAUDAL

Figure 7-6. Longitudinal section of the pelvis, demonstrating the urethra of the dog.

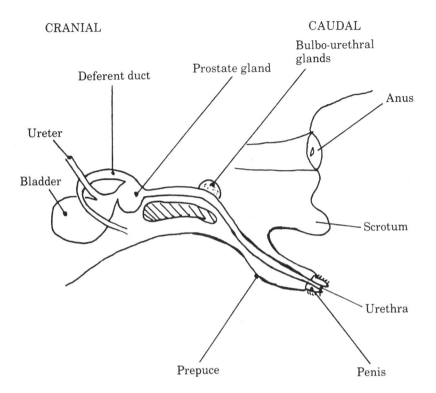

CRANIAL   CAUDAL

Bulbo-urethral glands

Prostate gland

Deferent duct

Anus

Ureter

Bladder

Scrotum

Urethra

Prepuce   Penis

Figure 7-7. Longitudinal section of the pelvis, demonstrating the urethra of the male cat.

an overlying fold of skin called the prepuce. This is continuous dorsally with the skin covering the caudal abdominal wall. The prepuce has an opening (the preputial orifice) in it through which the penis can protrude (as occurs at mating).

Catheterisation of the dog's bladder is easier than catheterising the bitch, but again a knowledge of regional anatomy is vital if this is to be performed safely. The dog should be restrained in lateral recumbency, with the uppermost hindleg retracted (by an assistant). The penis is extruded through the preputial orifice, the external urethral orifice is identified and a sterile lubricated catheter is carefully introduced into the urethra. Resistance to passage of the catheter tip may be met around the ischial arch, due to the bending of the urethra at this level. The catheter should never be forced, but the tip can be directed at this point by pressure applied either through the overlying skin, or by means of a gloved finger introduced into the rectum.

Although the urethra is a fibromuscular tube and is able to dilate to a certain degree, there are areas of potential narrowing where it may become obstructed due to the presence of urinary calculi (or stones). The first is the ischial arch where the urethra curves ventrally and is surrounded, in part, by

85

the pelvic bone. The second site is within the penis itself where the urethra runs ventral to the os penis; again a neighbouring boney structure limits the distensibility of the urethra. Urinary calculi form when concentrated urine comes into contact with damaged mucous membrane or when chemical changes, e.g. pH, makes its solutes less soluble – this easily happens with urinary infections. The price paid for efficient water conservation, i.e. concentrated urine, is that it may normally be close to the limit of solubility.

In the tom cat (Fig. 7-7) the urethra is short compared with that of the dog. It runs caudally on the floor of the pelvis and passes through the prostate gland. Continuing caudally, the urethra is next surrounded by the pair of bulbo-urethral glands (accessory sex glands). The urethra then passes caudo-ventrally to enter the penis (which lies just ventral to the scrotum). The urethra ends at the external urethral orifice. As the urethra runs caudally its internal diameter becomes progressively smaller, so obstruction (by urinary calculi) is most common at the caudal or penile urethra.

CHAPTER 8:
GASTROINTESTINAL SYSTEM AND DIGESTION

INTRODUCTION

Anatomically, the gastrointestinal system is a long tubular structure, running from the mouth to the anus. Food normally passes in one direction only and en route is subject to a variety of physical and chemical processes which bring about the digestion of food. It is logical to consider the anatomy of the gastrointestinal system by following the passage of food along it.

THE MOUTH

This is the first section of the gastrointestinal system, and its margins (or boundaries) are:

1. Laterally, the cheeks;

2. Dorsally, the palate;

3. Ventrally, muscles which lie below the tongue.

Caudally the mouth is continuous with the pharynx.

The cheeks are composed of muscles and an animal can consciously alter the position of the cheeks. Such movements are manifest as facial expression, a good example being a dog "snarling" in response to an aggressor. The inner surface is lined by mucous membrane.

The palate is divided into two sections. The hard palate is situated more rostrally and is supported by the overlying maxilla and palatine bones, hence it is firm and non-mobile with respect to neighbouring structures. The mucous membrane of the hard palate is thrown into several firm ridges, and may in part be pigmented. Caudally, the hard palate is continuous with the soft palate; this is composed of muscular tissue overlain by a smooth mucous membrane. The soft palate is quite mobile, and plays an important role in swallowing.

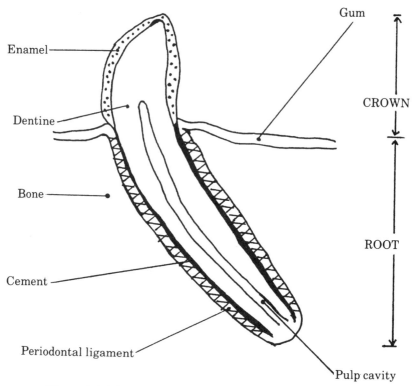

Figure 8-1. Diagram to show the structure of a canine tooth.

Within the mouth are the teeth which serve an important role in obtaining, cutting and crushing food (chewing or 'mastication'). It is as well to remember at this stage that both the dog and cat are carnivores and the shape and size of their teeth has evolved to allow them to obtain food "in the wild". It is only recently that these animals have been domesticated and been fed on specially prepared food, be it from a tin or packet! Teeth are exceptionally hard, and their roots are firmly positioned in special holes (called alveoli) in the jaw bones. Both the upper jaw bone (the maxilla) and the lower jaw bone (the mandible) are covered by the gum (or gingiva), the surface of which is continuous with the mucous membrane lining the cheeks and the palate. The section of a tooth which lies above the gum (i.e. the part which you see when examining an animal's mouth) is called the crown; that part below the gum (i.e. within the alveolus) is called the root.

A closer examination of a tooth's structure reveals a central pulp cavity which contains a soft, almost gel-like material called pulp (Fig. 8-1). The size of the pulp cavity (with respect to the size of the tooth) reduces as the animal gets older. The pulp cavity is surrounded by dentine, a hard material whose chemical composition and physical structure is not unlike that of bone. At the crown of the tooth, the dentine is covered by a layer of enamel. This is a very hard material, which enables the teeth to be used for physically breaking up food. At the root of a tooth, the dentine is covered by a thin layer of cement. The cement layer is joined to the bone around the alveolus by the periodontal ligament which is composed of a large number of interlocking strands of fibrous tissue. If this ligament is destroyed (e.g. by infection) then the tooth is no longer held firmly and may fall out.

Based upon their shape and position within the mouth, one can identify four basic types of teeth, all of which have different roles.

1. **The Incisors**
   These are situated at the front of the mouth. They have relatively small crowns with a sharp cutting surface. They serve to grasp and tear food.

2. **The Canines**
   These are very well developed in carnivores. The crowns are pointed so making them ideal for piercing food.

3. **The Premolars**

4. **The Molars**
   Premolars and molars together are often referred to as "cheek teeth". They are large teeth situated caudal to the canines, and usually have multiple roots (up to three per tooth). Their crowns have several projections or "cusps" which provide numerous sharp edges, used for cutting and crushing food. In the dog, the fourth upper premolar and the first lower molar are larger than the surrounding teeth; they are called the carnassial teeth and play an important role in cutting or crushing food.

Dental disorders commonly require treatment in veterinary practice, and an understanding of the basic disease processes is important. A common finding is the deposition of a film of bacteria, called plaque, on the surface of the crown. Before long, calcium salts, from the animal's saliva, are laid down on the plaque to form a firm layer, usually brown in colour, called dental calculus. Calculus is abrasive and its presence leads to the inflammation of the surrounding gum, a disease called gingivitis. In animals with gingivitis the gums appear reddened and swollen, and there is often bad breath (called halitosis). As the gums swell they lose their normal close contact with the surface of the crown, and this allows bacteria to start to destroy the periodontal ligament. As was stated earlier, destruction of this ligament leads to loosening of the tooth, and finally to tooth loss. It can be appreciated from this brief outline of the disease process that regular removal of plaque and dental calculus (often performed by using an ultrasonic descaling machine) is necessary to prevent gingivitis occurring.

Infection can reach the base of a tooth if there has been fracture of the crown, with exposure of the pulp cavity; infection spreads down the cavity leading to abscess formation at the tooth root. The infection may next track from the tooth root, through the surrounding bone, and discharge by means of a sinus tract to the overlying skin.

Destruction of the enamel layer of a tooth by acids produced by bacteria in the mouth causes the formation of holes or caries. This is a very common problem in human dentistry (usually associated with eating too much refined sugar), and most of us have required treatment for this problem by means of an amalgam filling placed within the hole. By contrast, this problem is not common in the dog, and exceptionally rare in the cat. If it does occur, then it may allow infection to occur in the underlying pulp cavity.

A characteristic of the mammals is that they possess two sets of teeth during their lifetime. In puppies the first (or deciduous) teeth erupt (their crowns being exposed in the mouth) from three weeks of age. The first set of teeth comprises only incisors, canines and premolars. In general, the deciduous teeth are similar to the permanent teeth, except they are smaller and sharper. At about three months of age, the deciduous teeth start to be lost, and are replaced by the permanent or second teeth. Normally all deciduous teeth will have been replaced by nine months of age. In certain smaller breeds of dog (e.g. Yorkshire Terriers) the deciduous teeth are not always lost, despite the permanent teeth erupting; this leads to a double row of teeth, with subsequent crowding and poor alignment of the permanent teeth. In such cases, it is necessary to remove the retained deciduous teeth.

The tongue is a thick muscular structure lying ventrally within the mouth. It is very mobile, and its dorsal surface feels roughened due to the presence of numerous projections or papillae; these are most noticeable on the cat's tongue. The "rasping" effect of the papillae is used when feeding, it is also used for grooming the animal's fur. The lingual artery and vein run on the ventral surface of the tongue. It is possible to monitor the peripheral pulse in the anaesthetised animal by palpating the lingual artery; one should not attempt to do this in the conscious patient!

The sense of taste (also called gustation), like the sense of smell, is well developed in dogs and cats. The receptors are inside taste buds which are situated close to the papillae of the tongue, and they are also found in the mucous membrane of the hard and soft palates (Chapter 11).

Saliva is a fluid secreted by the salivary glands in response to the presence of food within the mouth; however it can also be produced in anticipation of an animal being fed. The role of saliva in the carnivore is to lubricate the food, so allowing it to be swallowed easily; any enzymes present have an insignificant role in digestion (unlike human saliva).

There are four pairs of salivary glands (Fig. 8-2), situated close to the mouth. In addition, there are numerous small aggregates of salivary tissue actually within the mucous membrane lining the mouth. Saliva produced in the major salivary glands passes along small ducts to flow into the mouth.

The four pairs of 'major' salivary glands are:

1. **Parotid** gland; situated close to the external ear canal,

2. **Zygomatic** gland; situated just ventral to the eye,

3. **Submandibular** gland; situated close to the caudal edge of the mandible,

4. **Sublingual** gland; situated just ventral to the tongue.

Dogs and cats are often indiscriminate in what they eat, their menu ranging from the contents of the household dustbin (including plastic bags!) to their

90

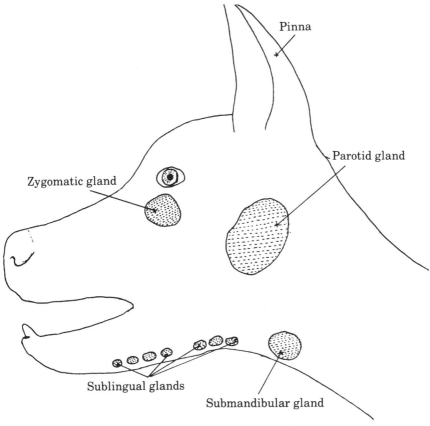

Figure 8-2. The salivary glands.

own or even other animal's faeces. The potential for introducing infection into the body by this route is obviously very high, and there is a need for surveillance and protection. For this reason there is an abundance of lymphoid tissue along the length of the gastrointestinal tract, and the mouth is no exception. The paired (i.e. left and right) tonsils are composed of lymphoid tissue, and are situated in the walls of the pharynx, caudal to the molar teeth. They normally lie in small recesses (or crypts) in the wall of the pharynx, and are not easily seen when examining a conscious animal. If there is infection within the mouth, the tonsils enlarge and protrude from the crypts, and are easily seen on oral examination. The tonsils may, in certain conditions, enlarge to such an extent as to interfere with normal functioning of the mouth and pharynx. Lymphoid tissue is also diffusely distributed in the mouth, within the hard and soft palates.

SWALLOWING

Food which has been broken down into small pieces as a result of mastication must next be swallowed. Swallowing is a complex process whereby a bolus (or ball) of food is propelled from the mouth back into the pharynx, and then on

1) Normal breathing.

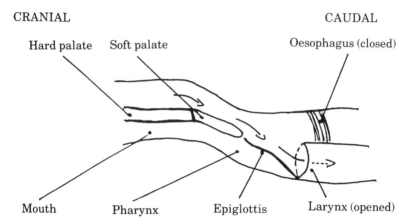

CRANIAL   CAUDAL

Hard palate   Soft palate   Oesophagus (closed)

Mouth   Pharynx   Epiglottis   Larynx (opened)

2) Swallowing

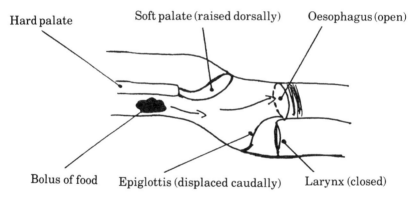

Hard palate   Soft palate (raised dorsally)   Oesophagus (open)

Bolus of food   Epiglottis (displaced caudally)   Larynx (closed)

Figure 8-3. Diagram to show the mechanisms of swallowing.

into the oesophagus. The bolus is moved by the tongue which acts as a 'plunger' combined with contraction of muscles in the wall of the pharynx. The pharynx is 'shared' by both the respiratory and gastrointestinal systems, so when swallowing the soft palate is raised (preventing food from passing into the nasal cavities), and the entrance to the larynx is closed (preventing food from passing down the trachea). At the same time, muscles which surround the entrance to the oesophagus relax, so allowing the bolus to enter (Fig. 8-3).

THE OESOPHAGUS

The oesophagus is a distensible, muscular tube which runs from the pharynx down to the stomach. The first (or cervical) section lies in the neck, close to the trachea. The second (or thoracic) section lies in the mediastinum within the

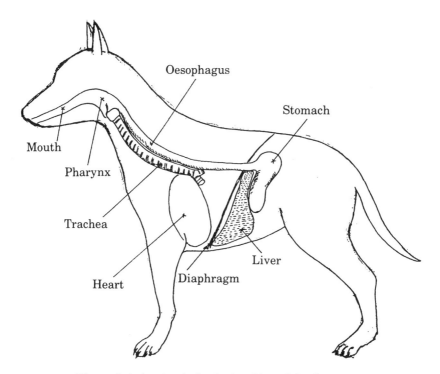

Figure 8-4. Anatomical relationships of the Oesophagus.

chest, and passes dorsal to the trachea and the heart. The thoracic oesophagus passes through a small opening (called a hiatus) within the diaphragm to enter the abdominal cavity, where it joins the stomach (Fig. 8-4).

Food moves along the oesophagus by means of peristalsis which involves the co-ordinated contraction of muscles within the oesophageal wall. In some animals the muscles of the oesophagus fail to function correctly, and there is inefficient peristalsis. This leads to the condition of megaoesophagus in which the oesophagus dilates along its length and food, once swallowed, fails to pass along to the stomach. It is then not uncommon for food to be returned to the mouth from the oesophagus when the head is lowered, for example when the animal is asleep. Megaoesophagus may be a congenital problem (i.e. present at birth) or may be acquired later in life.

THE STOMACH

The stomach is a thick-walled, sac-like structure, situated in the cranial section of the abdominal cavity, lying predominantly on the left side. Food enters from the oesophagus which joins the stomach at the cardia (Fig. 8-5). The entrance to the stomach is controlled by the cardiac sphincter and the exit by the pyloric sphincter.

The stomach is easily distended by its contents, and one of its main roles is to act as a reservoir for food. Again one must refer to the behaviour of carnivores

93

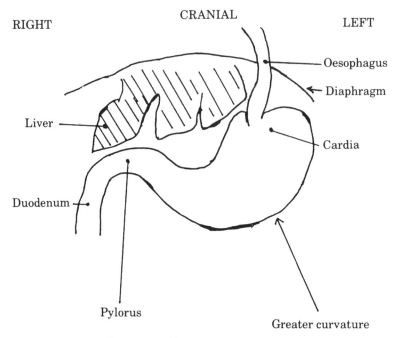

RIGHT CRANIAL LEFT

Oesophagus

Diaphragm

Liver

Cardia

Duodenum

Pylorus

Greater curvature

Figure 8-5. The stomach.
(Viewed from ventral aspect)

in the wild where they may only eat one very large meal every three or four days. At this time they attempt to eat as much food as they can (knowing that any left behind will will be eaten by another animal, and certainly would not be there on the following day!), thereby filling the stomach. The food is then slowly digested and small amounts are allowed to pass into the small intestines. Puppies often have ravenous appetites, and tend to eat so much food as to cause marked distension of the stomach which then presses on the overlying abdominal wall. In large breeds of dog (e.g. Great Danes) the stomach may dilate with gas, and then rotate on itself, occluding both its entrance and exit. This is the condition of "gastric dilatation and volvulus"; the exact cause is unclear, but the condition is one of the true life-threatening emergencies seen in veterinary practice.

The stomach wall is composed of an inner mucous membrane (or mucosa) supported on the underlying submucosal layer. Outside this the wall is made up of three layers of smooth (or visceral) muscle; their contraction leads to the mixing of ingesta within the stomach. The lining layer of the stomach, called the gastric mucosa, is arranged in numerous folds (or rugae) which become flattened when the stomach is distended with food. Glands within the gastric mucosa produce hydrochloric acid plus the enzyme pepsin. The hydrochloric acid renders the stomach contents acidic; this will kill many harmful bacteria which have been swallowed with the food. In addition, pepsin (which initiates enzymic digestion of proteins) functions most efficiently in an acidic environment. The presence of acid and pepsin in the stomach could lead to

94

breakdown of the stomach wall itself, since this, like all other tissues of the body, is made up of numerous protein molecules. This process of "autodigestion" is prevented by the secretion of a protective layer of mucus by the gastric glands.

The end result of the mechanical and chemical digestive processes occurring in the stomach is formation of a soup-like fluid called chyme. Chyme leaves the stomach through the pylorus and passes into the duodenum (the first section of the small intestine). Chyme is moved by peristalsis; however, this must be combined with relaxation of a ring of smooth muscle (the pyloric sphincter) lying around the pylorus. The process of peristalsis, combined with relaxation of the pyloric sphincter is controlled by both chemical and nervous signals, and we are usually quite oblivious to it happening inside ourselves. In some animals the pylorus may fail to open correctly; this may be the result of an obstructing foreign body (e.g. a ball) or due to failure of the pyloric sphincter to relax adequately (seen in pyloric stenosis). The failure of chyme to pass into the duodenum invariably leads to the animal returning the gastric contents to the mouth; this is the process of vomiting.

THE INTESTINES

The intestines are the major site for enzymatic digestion of food and the subsequent absorption of the end-products; primarily this involves the small intestine. The intestine is a tubular structure which runs from the pylorus to the anus, and is supported within the abdominal cavity by a thin sheet of peritoneum called the mesentery. In the dog, the total length of intestine is about four times the animal's body length; this is accommodated in the abdomen by being folded upon itself.

The intestines may be divided into two major regions according to their diameter. The small intestine is the proximal, or first section of the intestine, and its diameter is, as its name suggests, less than that of the more distally sited large intestine. At the junction of the small and large intestine there is a small blind-ending sac, called the caecum.

THE SMALL INTESTINE

The mucosa of the small intestine is composed of a large number of microscopic finger-like projections called villi (singular; villus). The presence of villi dramatically increases the effective surface area of the intestine in contact with ingesta, and increases the efficiency of digestion and absorption.

Ingesta move along the intestines by peristalsis, which involves the co-ordinated contraction of smooth muscle within the intestinal wall. It is not uncommon for there to be noise (borborygmi) associated with movement of ingesta by peristalsis: this "rumbling" within the abdomen may be heard by auscultation with a stethoscope.

Lying within the mesentery of the small intestine are numerous collections of lymphoid tissue. They play an important role in ensuring that any pathogens (disease-causing organisms) which may penetrate the intestinal wall are

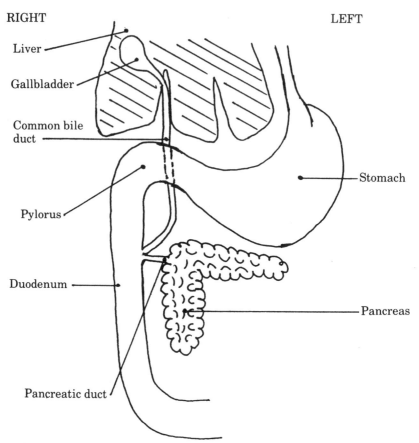

RIGHT   LEFT

Liver

Gallbladder

Common bile
duct

Stomach

Pylorus

Duodenum

Pancreas

Pancreatic duct

Figure 8-6. Diagram to show position of duodenum, and neighbouring structures.
(Viewed from ventral aspect).

trapped and destroyed. If an animal is suffering from an infection within the intestine (e.g. canine parvovirus) it is common for the lymphoid tissue to respond by becoming swollen and enlarged.

The small intestine is divided into three sections:

1. The **duodenum**

2. The **jejunum**

3. The **ileum.**

The Duodenum

The first section of the small intestine, starting at the pylorus. It is quite short, and is relatively non-mobile within the abdomen (compared with the later sections of the small intestine) being supported by a short mesentery.

96

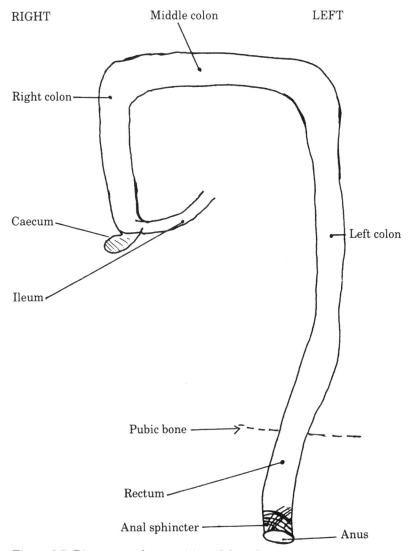

RIGHT   Middle colon   LEFT

Right colon

Caecum

Ileum

Left colon

Pubic bone ——→

Rectum

Anal sphincter

Anus

Figure 8-7. Diagram to show position of the colon.
(Viewed from ventral aspect, stomach and small intestine removed for clarity).

Intestinal glands situated at the base of the villi produce secretions which contain a variety of enzymes needed for digestion. In addition, enzymes produced at the pancreas (which lies within the mesentery supporting the duodenum) pass into the duodenal lumen via the pancreatic duct (Fig. 8-6). All these enzymes function most efficiently in an alkaline environment which is provided by the secretion of bicarbonate ions from the duodenum and pancreas. Bile (produced in the liver) also enters the duodenum, where it acts rather like washing-up liquid, to emulsify (or break up) fats.

The Jejunum

This is composed of numerous coils of intestine supported by mesentery. At this site the mesentery is relatively long and the jejunum is quite mobile within the abdomen. For the same reason, the jejunum is easily exteriorised from the abdomen at the time of laparotomy. In the more proximal sections of the jejunum the digestion of food predominates, but as one passes distally along it absorption (both of electrolytes, and the products of digestion) prevails.

The Ileum

The terminal section of the small intestine, which joins to the colon (or large intestine) is the ileum and its primary function is the absorption of electrolytes (mineral salts) and products of digestion.

THE LARGE INTESTINE

The large intestine is composed of the colon and the caecum. Compared with the small intestine, the colon wall appears thicker, and, in the live animal, is slightly blue/grey in colour. The mesenteric attachments of the colon are shorter than those of the small intestine so the colon has a relatively "fixed" position within the abdomen.

The ileum joins the first section of the colon, called the right colon. This next turns through 90 degrees to become the middle colon. A second 90-degree turn leads into the left colon which passes caudally in the abdomen, and enters the pelvic cavity to terminate at the anus. The intra-pelvic section of the colon is called the rectum (Fig. 8-7).

The colon plays an important role in the absorption of both water and electrolytes from the remains of the ingesta, and by doing so, forms the waste product of digestion called faeces. To aid passage of the faeces, glands within the mucosa of the colon secrete mucus which acts as a lubricant.

The caecum is a blind sac attached to the right colon, close to the ileum: it is much less important than in herbivores where it serves a site of bacterial digestion of cellulose. In humans it reduces still further to purely nuisance value – the appendix.

THE RECTUM AND ANUS

The rectum is continuous with the skin at the anus, which is situated just ventral to the tail base. The anus is normally closed due to contraction of a ring of muscle called the anal sphincter. Upon defaecating, this spincter relaxes, and faeces stored in the rectum are forced out by:

1. Contraction of smooth muscle within the rectal wall

2. Contraction of the muscles of the abdominal wall, which raises the intra-abdominal and intra-pelvic pressures.

Normal defaecation is dependent upon the co-ordinated contraction of numerous muscles, and requires that their nerve supply is intact. Animals with a damaged spinal cord (e.g. following a road accident) may lose nervous control of defaecation, with subsequent retention of faeces in the colon.

Animals may experience difficulty in defaecating if structures close to the rectum enlarge and impinge upon it (e.g. the prostate gland). Similarly, a fractured pelvis may heal incorrectly, and the displaced bones press on the rectum, preventing normal defaecation, and leading to constipation.

Positioned on either side of the terminal rectum (at 4 o'clock and 8 o'clock, as viewed from behind the animal) and surrounded by the anal sphincter, are the anal sacs. These are lined by modified sebaceous glands which produce a foul-smelling fluid (at least to us!). The fluid is stored in the sacs, and is discharged to the rectum at the time of defaecation. The fluid released has a role in "territory" marking. Perhaps more important, from a veterinary viewpoint, is the problem of infection and impaction of the anal sacs which leads to severe anal irritation and pain.

THE LIVER

The liver, the largest organ in the body, is situated in the cranial section of the abdomen, next to the diaphragm, with the stomach and small intestines lying on its caudal surface. The liver is composed of several lobes. The gallbladder is a small, sac-like structure which lies on the liver's surface, between two of the lobes. Bile, produced by the liver cells, flows along a vast network of small ducts to enter into the gallbladder where it is stored and concentrated. Contraction of the gallbladder leads to expulsion of bile along the common bile duct, which enters the duodenum close to the opening of the pancreatic duct. Since bile is required for the digestion of fats it is not surprising to learn that emptying of the gallbladder is stimulated very effectively by the presence of fatty foods within the duodenum. The common bile duct is a fragile structure, and may be occluded by tumours arising in the surrounding tissues which expand and compress the duct. This will prevent the normal excretion of bile which, instead, will be resorbed into the bloodstream, and lead to the animal becoming jaundiced. Strangely, in horses, there is no gallbladder so bile passes directly from the liver to the duodenum.

THE PANCREAS

This is a small organ lying within the mesentery of the duodenum. It is normally salmon-pink in colour, and is seen to be composed of multiple lobules (i.e. small lobes) joined together (Fig. 8-6).

The exocrine function of the pancreas is responsible for secretion of enzymes and bicarbonate ions. Some dogs (and occasionally cats) fail to produce sufficient pancreatic enzymes; this leads to a failure of digestion, especially of fats. Undigested fats pass through to the large intestine and are excreted to the faeces which have a characteristic "rancid" smell. It is possible to treat this condition by providing the missing enzymes, either as a powder or tablet, in the food.

The second, and more important, function of the pancreas is the production of hormones needed for the control of blood glucose. Insulin is produced by the

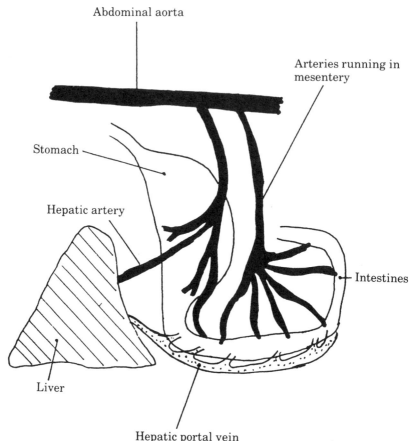

Abdominal aorta

Arteries running in
mesentery

Stomach

Hepatic artery

Intestines

Liver

Hepatic portal vein

Figure 8-8. Longitudinal section of the abdomen to demonstrate blood supply
of the gastrointestinal system.

Islets of Langerhans in the pancreas, and failure to manufacture adequate
amounts leads to the condition of diabetes mellitus (see below).

BLOOD SUPPLY OF THE GASTROINTESTINAL SYSTEM

The stomach, intestines, liver and pancreas all receive arterial blood from
branches of the abdominal aorta. This provides oxygen and nutrients needed
for cellular metabolism. The arteries reach the wall of the stomach and
intestine by travelling within the supporting mesentery.

The end-products of digestion, plus the large quantity of electrolytes and fluid
which are resorbed by the intestinal villi, pass into veins running in the wall
of the intestines. These veins lead directly to the liver, and make up the
hepatic portal venous system (Fig. 8-8). This allows the liver to monitor the

material absorbed from the intestines, rendering most toxic materials harmless; it may also trap and destroy any pathogens present in the blood. This system also gives the liver first access to the biologically useful products of digestion, many of which it requires to produce proteins and other substances needed by the body.

In summary, the liver has a dual blood supply from:

1. The hepatic artery, providing oxygen and some nutrients,
2. The hepatic portal vein, delivering the end-products of digestion.

Not all the products of digestion pass into the hepatic portal vein; the end-products of fat digestion are absorbed into the lacteals which make up part of the lymphatic system. Fats pass in the lymphatic system up through the thoracic duct to enter the cranial vena cava within the thorax.

THE ABDOMINAL CAVITY

Having discussed the arrangement of the gastrointestinal system, it is important that some consideration is given to the abdominal cavity itself. It is the largest of the body's cavities, and by comparison with the thorax, has a non-rigid wall.

The margins of the abdominal cavity are:

1. Cranially, the diaphragm;
2. Dorsally, the thoracic and lumbar vertebrae, with the associated sublumbar muscles;
3. Caudally, the pelvic cavity (the junction between the two being defined as the cranial limit of the pubic bone);
4. Laterally and ventrally, the muscular abdominal wall, plus, more cranially, the last three or four ribs.

The abdominal wall is largely composed of four pairs of muscles. The major part of the wall comprises three pairs of broad, flat sheets of muscle which originate from the lateral surface of the ribs, from the connective tissue and muscles surrounding the lumbar vertebrae and from the ilium (part of the bony pelvis). The muscles extend ventrally to meet their "opposite" number at the ventral midline (also called the linea alba). Situated more ventrally in the body wall there is a fourth muscle group (called the rectus abdominis) which lies on either side of the midline, and runs from the sternum and ribs to the pubis (Fig. 8-9).

The abdominal wall serves to:

1. Protect and support the abdominal contents.
2. Assist various bodily functions since contraction and relaxation of the muscles in the abdominal wall alters the pressure within the abdominal cavity. These functions include respiration, defaecation, urination and parturition (the process of giving birth).

101

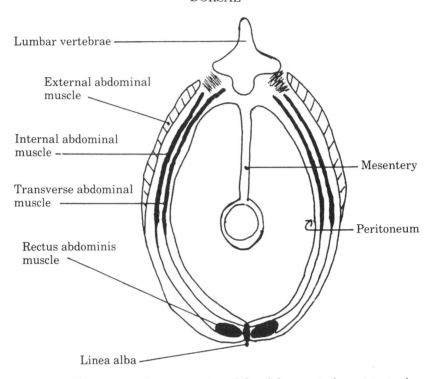

DORSAL

Lumbar vertebrae

External abdominal muscle

Internal abdominal muscle

Transverse abdominal muscle

Rectus abdominis muscle

Linea alba

Mesentery

Peritoneum

Figure 8-9. Diagrammatic cross-section of the abdomen, to demonstrate the structure of the abdominal wall.

Lining the inner surface of the abdominal wall is a thin membrane, called the peritoneum. This tissue lines the whole of the abdominal cavity and extends to cover the surface of intra-abdominal structures (e.g. the stomach and intestines). The mesentery, which supports the intestines from the dorsal wall of the abdomen, is also composed of peritoneum.

At a few sites there are small openings within the abdominal wall. Their function is to allow the passage of certain structures into and out of the abdomen. An example is the umbilicus which is an opening in the ventral midline which allows blood vessels to pass from the foetal abdomen to the placenta. In the region of the groin, lateral to the midline, is a slit-like opening in the muscles of the abdominal wall called the inguinal canal. In the male, the testes develop within the abdomen, but before long migrate out of the abdomen to reside in the scrotum. To reach this position they must pass through the inguinal canal, and in doing so they take their blood supply with them. Hence, in the adult male, dissection of the inguinal canal reveals that it contains the testicular artery and vein, and the deferent duct.

Both the umbilicus and the inguinal canal are classified as physiologically "normal" openings (although the umbilicus usually closes soon after birth).

102

Occasionally, these "normal" openings enlarge, usually due to weakness of the surrounding muscles; this may allow abdominal contents (e.g. intestines) to pass through the hole, leading to a clinically apparent swelling. This condition is a hernia whereas an **abnormal** opening in the abdominal wall is called a rupture.

To gain surgical access to the abdominal contents it is necessary to make an incision in the abdominal wall. A variety of surgical approaches are available, but broadly they can be divided into two categories.

1. Those where an incision is made in the ventral abdominal wall, either through the linea alba, or just to one side of it; or

2. An incision made in the lateral abdominal wall, a so-called "flank" approach. It is necessary to cut through the three layers of muscles making up the abdominal wall at this point. The flank approach is commonly used for ovarohysterectomy (speying) in the cat.

FEEDING, BEHAVIOUR AND DIGESTION

When we learn about digestion, in one sense, we learn about learning itself. We have all seen dogs literally drooling at the sight of cheese, apple, chocolate, whatever takes their fancy. This sight took the fancy of the great Russian scientist Pavlov who showed that this anticipation of good food could be stretched further until anything which the dog learned to associate with imminent feeding would provoke salivation. So a dog could be taught to salivate purely at the sound of a bell or the sight of a particular object if this was normally followed by feeding. In other words, a **reflex** response to food could be **conditioned** to become a reflex response to an entirely different stimulus. Many other reflexes can be 'conditioned' and, for example, a dog that is terrified of thunder may become conditioned to fear rain.

This is not the only type of conditioning. Animals can also be conditioned to produce behaviour not because it is a reflex but because they have learned that it produces a reward (or not to produce behaviour because it leads to pain or fear). This alternative to 'classical' conditioning is called operant conditioning and is quite obviously the basis of many animal training routines, most of them familiar long before scientists 'invented' operant conditioning. It is also an extremely useful way of asking animals whether they can discriminate between colours, shapes, sounds, etc. in order to obtain a reward. One of the strongest rewards is an attractive food.

Why begin a discussion of digestive function with behaviour? Because feeding, alongside sex and mothering, is probably the most important behaviour which animals indulge in; certainly, so far as we can be sure, it is one of their greatest pleasures. But this pleasure, this slobbering at the sight of the Sunday joint, has other vital yet mundane functions. Dogs do not spend much time chewing and savouring food; the better it is, the quicker they bolt it. So if saliva is to provide sufficient lubrication for swallowing it needs to be turned on in advance. This is simply one particularly vivid demonstration of a recurrent feature of digestion; mechanisms are activated in **anticipation** of the delivery of food or digesta, they do not simply await its arrival.

103

Animals learn – become conditioned – that certain aromas, tastes, are either rewarding in themselves or lead to pleasant sensations during digestion. Equally, they learn that certain tastes are associated with subsequent feelings of illness, and are best avoided. The protective potential of this response is obvious but this type of learning – bait shyness (learned aversion) – can also create problems. If a particular food is tainted or poisoned, or if a food is quite harmless but happens to be eaten just before acute illness the animal may become strongly conditioned to avoid it.

DIGESTION: GENERAL

The need to eat and digest food results from two inescapable obligations of life; to provide energy and to replenish tissues. The skin, hair, gut cells, blood cells we have at Christmas are almost none of them the ones we had at Easter: they are continuously being replaced. A great anatomist once pointed out the enigma of the constancy of the body's form with a vivid analogy; it is like the constancy of our image reflected in a flowing stream – there is no change in what we see yet the substance of the image is continually changing. That continuous replacement of tissue demands protein and our need for energy demands carbohydrate and fat. The younger the animal the greater the need in proportion to size in order to provide for growth, greater activity and greater heat loss through the greater surface area of a smaller size (Chapter 4).

Even the nature of the re-supply process is remarkable. There is little difference between the muscle of a dog or a sheep but when a dog eats meat and uses that protein to build or replenish muscle, it takes it apart down to the elementary building blocks – amino acids – within the gut and then, having absorbed them, reconstructs the protein all over again. This process of total breakdown to elementary units, absorption of these simple units and their utilisation to reconstruct protein, fat or carbohydrate is a striking characteristic of digestion. It substantially reflects the fact that the intestine has specific absorptive mechanisms for a relatively restricted repertoire of chemicals. In part this is protective – it helps to absorb preferentially what is safe and necessary.

Nevertheless, not all absorbed substances are broken down nor do they all need specific absorptive mechanisms. Some are simply absorbed because they are small enough and easily cross the intestinal wall. In some cases this is advantageous, e.g. vitamins and other nutrients would be damaged sufficiently to be unusable if they were first broken down. On the other hand, poisons may be absorbed in the absence of any special absorptive mechanisms. Water is also absorbed without a specific mechanism; it simply follows the osmotic gradient created by the active absorption of sodium (or other solutes).

The fact that digestion causes progressive dismantling of many substances means that some drugs cannot be given orally or they will be broken down – protein hormones like insulin are obvious examples. Other drugs may remain intact but fail to be absorbed, in which case they could still be useful within the gut, e.g. neomycin. For one unique period of life – the first few hours – the intestine is very permeable to proteins, allowing the protective antibodies in colostrum (first milk) to be absorbed, provided the newborn animal receives sufficient soon enough.

Perhaps the most fascinating aspect of digestion is the environment in which it occurs, the lumen of the gut itself. It is, literally, a special environment situated within the body yet not quite part of it. The gut contents have not yet crossed any cell membranes (except for the intestinal secretion). The gut is a direct continuation of the external environment. Like the lungs or the skin, therefore, it is a site of risk, a site where harmful substances or organisms could gain entry. The lungs are largely protected by the simplicity of their contents – air – and the arrangements in the upper respiratory tract and airways which filter or eject foreign particles (Chapter 3). Skin is protected partly by its thickness and the fact that the outer layer, the final protective contact, is dead and tough. But the gut contents provide the challenge of contaminated soil or plants, infected meat, jagged particles of bone yet ultimately they must be presented to a surface so delicate and richly supplied with blood that the essential nutrients are efficiently absorbed.

The intestine thus allows potentially hazardous contact between the internal and external environment. Protective mechanisms, as we shall see, are therefore a crucial aspect of digestive function. The gut cannot simply be thick and inert, like the epidermis, though it can share with skin the protection of its own harmless natural flora, or bacterial population. It is like a microscopic 'neighbourhood watch', keeping marauders at bay. Blasting the intestine indiscriminately with antibiotics to clear out pathogens (bacteria capable of causing disease) carries the same hazard as 'nuking' intruders in a neighbourhood; it may also destroy the normal population. The balances between useful bacteria and pathogens, physiology and disease are just as delicate in this environment as those in the ecology of the countryside. A few well intentioned chemicals can create a lot of unintended mischief.

PREHENSION, MASTICATION: MECHANICS OF DIGESTION

The logic of digestion is as simple as the plan which would be needed to convert a car back to pure iron, rubber and plastics. First we would need to dismantle it. Then we would need to break the chunks down to usable fragments. Finally we would need some clever chemistry. It would require a team and they would have to work in the right order; no use giving the chunks to the chemists until they are small enough and properly prepared.

A single logical sequence converts a chunk of beef down to the single amino acids which need to be absorbed. It begins with 'spanners and sledgehammers', with biting and chewing. It proceeds with the more delicate mechanical dismantling by the churning of the stomach and intestinal movements and it culminates in the precise splitting of one molecule from another by specific digestive enzymes. All the time the particle size is decreasing and the number of particles is increasing. As the particles get smaller the total surface area exposed to chemical attack gets larger. Digestion is remarkably fast. It would take a very sophisticated laboratory to match the few hours which it takes a dog to digest a chicken.

CHEMISTRY OF DIGESTION: ENZYMES

Enzymes are proteins which accelerate (catalyse) chemical reactions; they are **biological catalysts**. They are necessary for many reactions within the cells of all tissues. Their special importance in intestinal secretions is that they accelerate the breakdown of fat, carbohydrate and protein. Enzymes are also very specific; they attack a particular detail of chemical structure and no other. Their names often indicate the substances (**substrates**) on which they act, thus enzymes attacking lipids (fats) are lipases, those attacking sugars such as maltose or lactose are maltase and lactase, and cellular enzymes which liberate energy from ATP by splitting it down to ADP (Chapter 1) are ATPases.

In general the steps in dismantling proteins are: protein, to amino acid chains (polypeptides), to double amino acids, to single amino acids (peptides). Each step needs a different type of enzyme. The same is true of the carbohydrate sequence: carbohydrates, to double sugars (disaccharides), to single sugars (e.g. glucose). These progressive sequences take place as the intestinal contents (**chyme**) proceed along the gut and each region of the gut produces a different range of enzymes appropriate to the stage of breakdown at which it receives the digesta. Fats progressively break down to fatty acids and other simple lipid products. By the time the chyme reaches the absorptive areas of the gut it contains the simple sugars, such as glucose, simple amino acids and fatty acids which are ideal for absorption.

Not only must a region receive digesta at the accustomed stage of breakdown, it must have sufficient time for its own enzymes to work. Otherwise the next region will receive digesta prematurely, with breakdown incomplete, and its enzymes may not find the substrates which they are adapted to attack. If this happens, these substrates may accumulate and allow alien bacteria to flourish which would not survive in more normal surroundings. A similar thing may occur if an animal is unable to produce its usual enzymes, either because of a genetic defect or during recovery from intestinal disease. The accumulating substrates will also trap water, osmotically, and some may be irritant or act as local poisons. We thus have the setting for diarrhoea without any need to 'pick up a germ'.

The intestine is accustomed to producing a particular range of enzymes suited to the normal variety of foods. Some adaptation and readjustment is possible in the event of a major dietary change, but this takes time. Sudden changes of diet can disrupt digestion by presenting new substrates for which the current range of enzymes is not ideally suited. Again, substrates may stay in a form unsuited for absorption and this **'malabsorption'** will cause diarrhoea. Neither bacteria, nor viruses nor intestinal inflammation (enteritis) are necessary for the occurrence of diarrhoea. An inappropriate or suddenly altered diet is a very common cause; this, rather than unclean food or water probably underlies most 'holiday diarrhoea'. Sudden changes of diet have another harmful effect – they may produce an unfavourable environment for the normal bacterial flora without allowing it time to adapt or change.

SECRETIONS: DIARRHOEA

Each region of the gut produces its own characteristic secretions and others are added by the pancreas and liver. It is important that the secretions not only carry enzymes but also ensure that the region has the appropriate acidity (pH) to allow its enzymes to work; enzymes are very 'choosy' about their ideal ('optimum') pH. Thus the acidity of the gastric secretions is neutralised by the strongly alkaline pancreatic secretion which is added in the duodenum.

Secretions also provide lubrication, notably saliva and gastric secretion because at this stage the food is still coarse and abrasive compared with the smoother consistency of chyme. Mucus is also an important lubricant in intestinal secretions, notably in the large intestine, especially the colon, where the contents become drier as water is salvaged and the characteristic faeces are formed.

All the way from the mouth to the colon there is a tremendous outpouring of secretions – not just when food or digesta arrive but in anticipation, induced either psychologically (saliva and gastric secretions) or reflexly, triggered from the preceding region or by local hormones. Saliva is a very watery secretion in dogs and, unlike human saliva, it has no digestive enzymes. Intestinal secretions are rich in salts (sodium, potassium, chloride and bicarbonate) all of which must be retrieved along with water further along the intestine in order to be 'recycled'. Thus most of the sodium absorbed in the intestine comes not from the diet but from the animal's own secretions. The **final** salvage of sodium and water is a crucial function of the colon.

When sodium absorption fails, water also accumulates in the intestinal contents and eventually they may overwhelm the colon's ability to intensify its salt and water conservation. The faeces then become liquid; the animal has diarrhoea. Apart from the inconvenience, it loses potentially dangerous amounts of water, sodium, potassium and bicarbonate. If fat digestion fails the faeces may be fatty and rancid, whether or not there is diarrhoea.

Obviously the treatment of diarrhoea is two-fold. One is to treat the cause or to help the animal to overcome it. If it is severe, however, it becomes vital to prevent serious sodium depletion, dehydration and acidosis (bicarbonate loss; Chapter 7) by fluid therapy. Above all, this must replace the lost sodium (osmotic skeleton) if ECF volume is to be restored, and circulatory collapse prevented.

Traditionally fluid therapy has been intravenous, and still needs to be if shock has occurred. Recently, however, all but the severest diarrhoeas have been tackled by oral rehydration, an approach based on the treatment of human cholera (still one of the acutest diarrhoeas and the most prevalent in poor countries). Since diarrhoea is fundamentally either a failure of sodium and water reabsorption or an abnormal secretory accumulation it seems strange to add even more sodium to the animal's intestine. The key lies in the ability of solutions with a particular composition (or something close to it) to increase sodium uptake despite the underlying disease. Not every diarrhoea responds but a remarkable variety do. The 'magic' solution has the same osmotic

107

concentration as plasma (i.e. it is isotonic, Chapter 5) and has equal concentrations of sodium and glucose (in mmol/l, not mg/l). In simple terms this means something like 100 mmol/l Na^+ and 2% glucose. The glucose is not there to provide energy (it provides very little at that concentration) but to promote sodium uptake. Certain amino acids such as glycine and fatty acid salts such as citrate or acetate further assist the absorption of sodium from these 'oral rehydration solutions' (ORS). It is said that they may save more human lives than antibiotics and they have been extensively used in calf diarrhoea and canine parvoenteritis. Their success emphasises that what kills animals with diarrhoea is usually neither infection nor gut damage but dehydration, loss of circulating volume and acidosis.

The fluid loss leading to clinically obvious dehydration in diarrhoea is plainly visible. It may be more puzzling that intestinal obstruction, with no apparent losses, can also lead to dehydration, shock, and the need for fluid therapy. In this case, however, the fluid accumulates within swollen and damaged gut as a result of oversecretion, absorptive failure and capillary damage. This abnormal accumulation of fluid may still be in the animal but it is not where it is needed, i.e. in ECF and plasma in particular. Moreover distension of the gut (not only by fluid but by gas released by fermentation) makes capillary damage increasingly likely, accompanied by further fluid loss; a vicious cycle which can rapidly lead to shock (Chapter 6). Twisting of the gut (or stomach) causes a similar sequence, not only by obstructing it but by blocking venous circulation (hence raising capillary pressure and causing further fluid loss) or even arterial circulation (leading to cell death (necrosis) and further deterioration).

DIGESTION IN SPECIFIC GUT REGIONS

Having discussed the general features of digestion and some aspects of digestive disturbances it is necessary to consider some more specific aspects in relation to each gut region and the movement of food between them. In addition we have to understand the importance of two organs which work in close conjunction with the gut; the liver and pancreas.

MOUTH: SWALLOWING: VOMITING

The teeth and salivary glands fragment and moisten the food, ready for swallowing. Touch your throat below the 'Adam's apple': you can feel the trachea – obviously it is in front of your oesophagus. Yet your nasal passages clearly lead behind your mouth. So the airway and the food path cross over and (apart from sound production) the vital function of the larynx is to close the trachea during swallowing. Food does not fall down the oesophagus to the stomach by gravity; if it did veterinary students would be unable to drink beer standing on their heads and astronauts would have even more problems. Instead the food is propelled by waves of muscular contraction, like a self-squeezing toothpaste tube. This type of movement, 'peristalsis', is found throughout the intestine. Peristaltic waves can abnormally run backwards, as they do in vomiting, and this can happen in any region of the gut. Thus vomit can be stained by bile although bile does not normally enter the stomach.

Vomiting is triggered by gastrointestinal irritation and also by a special area in the brain hence it can be caused by drugs, non-gastrointestinal disease, travel sickness, etc. Although antiperistalsis may return intestinal contents to the stomach as a prelude to vomiting the main force is finally the contraction of the diaphragm and abdominal muscles, with the cardiac sphincter relaxed. In moderation vomiting is an excellent protective response because it rejects food which may be poisoned or contaminated, before it can reach the absorptive areas of the gut.

STOMACH

The stomach stores the meal, acidifies it to kill potential pathogens, mixes its contents and continues mechanical breakdown of the food. It initiates chemical digestion by adding enzymes and liberates its contents in an orderly fashion over a period of time, when they are sufficiently prepared to be received by the duodenum. The gastric contractions which mix the food do not empty the stomach because it is closed at its entrance and exit by sphincters – rings of muscle. These relax during swallowing (cardiac sphincter) or emptying (pyloric sphincter).

DUODENUM

The duodenum receives chyme from the stomach and adds pancreatic secretions. These are very alkaline and neutralise the gastric acid. They also contain enzymes to continue the breakdown of protein, fat and carbohydrate; these enzymes have an alkaline optimum pH. The duodenum also receives the secretion of the liver, bile, which is stored and concentrated in the gall bladder. It provides an additional excretory route used by many drugs, and by bile pigments, the end product of the breakdown of haemoglobin from exhausted red cells. The bile pigments colour the faeces and if their flow is obstructed, faeces become pale but the animal becomes yellow (jaundiced) as the pigments accumulate in circulation.

The other essential contribution of bile is to provide bile salts which act like detergents to emulsify fats, i.e. break them up into minute particles which are more susceptible to attack by the fat digesting enzymes (lipases). Thus although bile contains no enzymes it is essential for the effective action of the pancreatic enzymes in fat digestion. Failure of pancreatic secretion or of liver function results in poor digestion and absorption of fat and may cause fatty faeces (steatorrhoea). Disturbances of fat absorption may also prevent the absorption of fat-soluble vitamins.

JEJUNUM AND ILEUM

The bulk of the small intestine consists of the jejunum and ileum. It is highly active, with segmenting movements which mix the secretions into the chyme and propulsive movements which continue its progress towards the large intestine. These movements are co-ordinated by local nerve networks (plexuses) in the intestinal wall and produced by its longitudinal and circular layers of smooth muscle (Chapter 12). The surface area for secretion is increased by the intestinal **crypts** and the surface area for absorption is increased by the finger-like **villi**. Naturally, if the gut and its capillaries become damaged, this large surface area becomes a dangerously effective route of fluid loss. The fluid may still be within the body but it is no longer where it is needed, in circulation.

The lifespan of intestinal cells is extremely short, a few days, i.e. the turnover of replacement and loss into the lumen is rapid. As the cells mature they migrate towards the tips of the villi and as they migrate their secretory capacity matures. Enteric disease easily disrupts this migration and the result can be an astonishingly rapid flattening of the intestinal villi and loss of both mature secretory cells and absorptive surface area. This adds to the underlying problem and since restoration of villous structure takes time, resumption of a normal diet may not be immediately acceptable even though recovery from the original disturbance is satisfactory.

The intestinal juices add enzymes which are specific for smaller and smaller chains of amino acids or sugars and fat digestion also continues. Absorption begins alongside digestion and many substances are absorbed along most of the small intestine. This is fortunate because it means that surgical removal (resection) of damaged intestine need not interfere with overall function. In any case there is some compensatory growth of the intestine beyond the resected area. Some substances, however, may only be absorbed within a restricted length of the intestine in which case seemingly minor damage may have considerable impact. One example is the bile salts. Even during digestion of a single meal they are secreted, reabsorbed and recycled. Reabsorption occurs only in a relatively small area of the ileum which, therefore, becomes essential for normal fat digestion.

The harmful effects of overactivity on intestinal function have already been described, with digesta arriving prematurely at the next region of the gut. Underactivity, especially complete stasis, can be equally damaging. Secretions may accumulate because they are upstream of their normal reabsorptive site. The bacterial flora may change unfavourably because alien bacteria instead of experiencing a constant succession of different environments, may have the chance to settle in one that suits them, or even adhere to the intestinal wall. The combination of substrate accumulation and a possibly abnormal flora allows fermentation to occur and to produce gas. This distends the gut and may inflict sufficient injury to cause leakage of fluid from circulation into the lumen, via damaged capillaries. The additional fluid intensifies the distension, thus establishing a vicious circle. The end results may include severe intestinal damage, depletion of circulatory volume (leading to shock) and almost certainly pain.

The problem may spread because pain in one area of the intestine can reflexly alter the activity of other regions. Normally this type of 'communication' between gut regions is useful in turning on anticipatory secretion or turning off activity in preceding areas once the main flow of chyme has passed. It is not only a matter of reflexes but of a number of local hormones, for example those produced in the stomach and intestine which control pancreatic secretion (gastrin, secretin, cholecystokinin).

Most of the digestive products absorbed from the intestine reach the hepatic portal vein, though those of fat digestion are substantially removed by the lymphatics. The significance of the hepatic portal vein is that it leads directly

110

to the liver allowing this organ first access to the various nutrients, as befits an organ with such a central role in the regulation of metabolism. A 'portal' vein is one which allows blood to travel directly from the capillaries of one tissue to those of another without first returning to the heart. The hepatic portal vein is the only major example in mammals (though a small portal system exists between the hypothalamus and the anterior pituitary gland).

LARGE INTESTINE

The large intestine of herbivores is extremely important in allowing them to use the bacteria in their normal flora to digest plant cell walls – something which mammalian enzymes cannot do. In dogs and cats its size and complexity is much reduced but the colon remains important in salvaging water and electrolytes from faeces, controlling their final sodium, potassium and water content. It also secretes mucus to lubricate them and allow easy movement despite their greater dryness.

LIVER

The liver is not only the largest organ in the body, it has a list of functions to match its size. In fulfilling them it uses a wide range of enzymes within its cells. Normally these enzymes are absent or undetectable in plasma but leakage from damaged cells can allow liver disease to be diagnosed from blood samples. The other main approach to the diagnosis of liver disease is to detect changes in one or other of the variety of hepatic functions. It has to be remembered, however, that the liver is not only large but, like the kidney, it has a substantial functional reserve capacity. In other words it can sustain a considerable amount of damage without showing signs of disease; many businessmen's lives depend on this!

The most important liver function is probably to stabilise blood glucose and this will be considered separately at the end. But the liver plays a central role in all aspects of metabolism. It has first access to the amino acids arriving from the intestine and it makes most of the blood proteins involved in

(i)   Clotting

(ii)   Nutrition

(iii) Transport of fats, hormones, iron, copper, calcium and magnesium.

In particular, it makes albumin and some of the globulins but it does not produce the immune globulins; these are produced by lymphocytes (Chapter 5).

The liver can also use amino acids to liberate energy and it can interconvert amino acids, i.e. produce those absent from dietary protein. Amino acids which cannot be produced in this way are 'essential' for that particular species of animal (e.g. taurine in cats). The liver is thus a vital organ in protein breakdown, either using the end products to form new amino acids or converting them via ammonia (which is very toxic) to urea which is relatively harmless and readily excreted in urine.

111

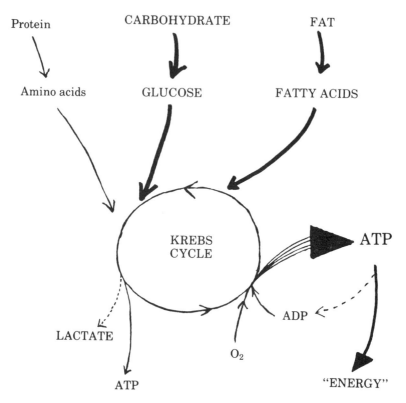

Figure 8-10. Conversion of food to energy (ATP).

When glucose is in short supply, the liver receives fatty acids mobilised from the body's fat depots and thus metabolises fat for energy. Conversely, when surplus carbohydrate (sugar) is available the liver converts it to fat which can be stored in liver or, more important, in fat depots, ready for leaner times.

As already explained (Chapters 3, 7) the liver is able to re-use any lactate accumulating from anaerobic metabolism; in doing so it supplies substrates for aerobic metabolism once the oxygen supply improves. These last, crucial steps of aerobic metabolism, which amplify the yield of ATP ten-fold, take place in the 'powerhouses' of the body cells, the mitochondria. The key step between the common preliminary pathway, supplying both aerobic and anaerobic metabolism, and the final stages in the mitochondria, is a complicated cycle of fatty acid interconversions (Kreb's cycle). Its main purpose is to supply substrates allowing the mitochondria to use oxygen to convert ADP to ATP (Fig. 8-10). The advantage of such a complex pathway, the details of which need not worry you, is to allow the final energy generators, the mitochondria, to be supplied indirectly from a variety of 'fuels' (glucose, fatty acids, even amino acids) derived when necessary from a variety of stores (carbohydrate, fat, even protein).

The fact that the liver is involved in so many apsects of energy metabolism makes it a major source of body heat (Chapter 4). It also produces the bile pigments (as end products of red cell breakdown) and bile salts (see above). The iron from red cell breakdown is substantially stored in the liver, ready for re-use. Obstruction to bile flow or abnormally increased production of bile pigment causes bile pigment to accumulate in circulation and to stain tissues yellow; the animal is 'jaundiced'. Excessive red cell breakdown (haemolysis) can obviously lead to jaundice, e.g. after a mismatched transfusion. This can either be a direct cause or it can sensitise the dam to the same blood group as some of her offspring. They then receive antibodies in colostrum which in this case are destructive instead of protective. Bile also serves as an excretory route for various normal metabolites, drugs and poisons and the liver converts many substances to a form which is readily eliminated from the circulation, either in bile or urine. The liver and kidneys are thus the major organs of excretion, with the lungs excreting CO_2.

The blood supply of the liver from the hepatic portal vein obviously makes it vulnerable to poisons and bacteria from the gut. Fortunately the liver is protected both by its detoxifying reactions and by scavenger cells (macrophages, Chapter 5). (Remember, the liver also has a conventional blood supply from the hepatic artery and a conventional venous drainage in the hepatic vein though within the liver the detailed vascular relationships are unusual.)

Finally we must return to the role of the liver in regulating blood glucose, a function shared with the pancreas.

LIVER, PANCREAS AND BLOOD GLUCOSE

The main role of the liver in the stabilisation of blood glucose is to act as a carbohydrate store, converting excess glucose to glycogen ('animal starch'). When blood glucose falls, the liver can liberate more glucose from glycogen, under the influence of hormones such as adrenaline, corticosteroids and glucagon. Hepatic glycogen stores only amount to an emergency supply, however, worth less than a day's total energy requirement. Long term inadequacy of dietary energy content can only be offset by drawing on fat depots.

The particular importance of regulating blood glucose between certain limits (it does vary acccording to meal pattern) is that the brain is extremely glucose-dependent unlike other tissues which can also utilise fatty acids. In fact brain is guaranteed 'first call' on the available glucose if plasma levels fall. This is because, unlike other tissues, it can take up glucose without the help of insulin. Since insulin is a post-absorptive hormone, helping cells to take up the glucose, amino acids and potassium resulting from the digestion of a meal, brain receives its preferential access precisely when insulin and glucose levels are both low, i.e. when further feeding has been delayed. If blood glucose falls too low to supply the brain the animal is likely to go into convulsions.

Blood glucose is regulated by two major feedback loops (as well as other hormones which need not concern us).

113

(a) A rise of blood glucose after a meal stimulates the release of insulin from the pancreas. This drives glucose into cells, helping them to utilise it, and corrects the rise of blood glucose (Fig. 8-11). The response corrects the disturbance; negative feedback (Chapter 1). Lack of insulin, or an inadequate response to it, is the common cause of diabetes mellitus with its abnormally high blood glucose.

(b) A fall of blood glucose not only reduces insulin secretion but causes the pancreas to secrete a different hormone, glucagon. This causes the liver to convert stored glycogen to glucose, correcting the fall in blood glucose; again, negative feedback.

The pancreas, like many areas of the intestine which produce local hormones, thus functions as both a conventional **exocrine gland** and an **endocrine gland.** These functions are served by different cell types within the gland. The distinction between exocrine and endocrine glands is that:

Exocrine glands produce secretions which are directed onto their targets by local ducts.

Endocrine glands produce secretions which travel usually to distant targets, sometimes to local targets, but always via the bloodstream, never via ducts.

These secretions are called hormones. The production and effects of hormones (endocrinology) are discussed further in the next Chapter.

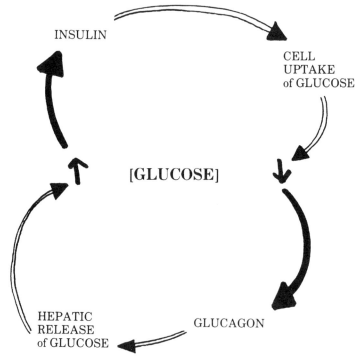

INSULIN

CELL
UPTAKE
of GLUCOSE

[GLUCOSE]

HEPATIC
RELEASE
of GLUCOSE

GLUCAGON

Figure 8-11. Regulation of blood glucose.

114

CHAPTER 9:
THE ENDOCRINE SYSTEM

The endocrine system is composed of numerous glandular organs, situated at various sites within the body (Fig. 9-1). They all produce chemical messengers (or hormones) which are secreted directly into the blood. The major role of the endocrine system is to control the body's internal environment and metabolism. A hormone, as we saw in the last chapter, is a specific secretion (from a gland) which travels to a distant tissue via the blood and there produces specific regulatory effects.

The basic control mechanism of the endocrine system is one of negative feedback; this has already been described in relation to the effects of insulin on blood glucose (Chapter 8). Indeed, because of the importance of hormones in controlling a variety of functions we have already learned about several, e.g. erythropoietin, aldosterone, ADH (Chapter 7), insulin and glucagon (Chapter 8). We have also learned the difference between exocrine and endocrine secretion, and the fact that some glands do both (Chapter 8).

It is a fair generalisation that we are usually unaware of the function of the endocrine system in the healthy animal (except for the effects of various sex hormones involved in reproduction). We become aware of hormonal function in cases of disease where the normal control mechanisms of secretion are, for one reason or another, rendered ineffective. Hence, in veterinary medicine we may be presented with an animal in which there is insufficient hormone production (this is given the prefix of "hypo-", e.g. hypothyroidism), or a situation in which there is an excessive production of hormone (given the prefix "hyper-", e.g. hyperthyroidism). In general terms, disorders of inadequate hormone production are treated by provision of exogenous hormone to the animal (usually by injection), whereas if there is excess hormone production this may, in some cases, be treated by the surgical removal of the "offending" gland. (Substances are 'exogenous' if they come from outside the body, 'endogenous' if they originate within.)

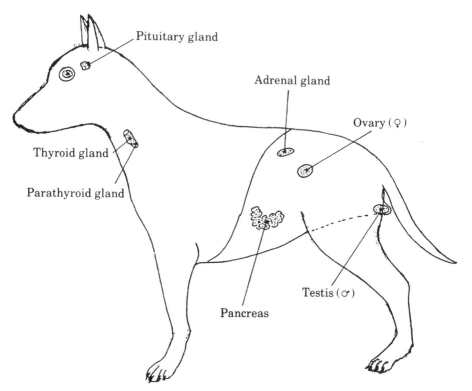

Figure 9-1. Major endocrine glands in the dog.

THE PITUITARY GLAND

The pituitary gland lies within the cranium, on the ventral surface of the midbrain, and is close to the region of the brain called the hypothalamus (Fig. 9-2). The pituitary plays an extremely important role in controlling the function of other endocrine glands. It is for this reason that the pituitary has been likened to the conductor of an orchestra, co-ordinating the numerous "musicians" represented by the endocrine glands.

Considering its small size, the pituitary gland is extremely versatile in producing a large number of hormones (Fig. 9-3).

Functionally, the pituitary may be divided into two areas:

1. The anterior pituitary

2. The posterior pituitary.

The hormones produced by the **anterior pituitary** are:

(1) **Thyroid Stimulating Hormone** (TSH)
   This acts on the thyroid glands, causing the production and release of thyroxine.

116

(2) **Adrenocorticotrophic Hormone** (ACTH)
ACTH acts on the adrenal cortex, and stimulates its growth, and the production and release of cortisol.

(3) **Growth Hormone** (GH, also called **Somatotropin**)
Growth hormone stimulates growth in a wide variety of the body's tissues, ranging from bone to mammary tissue. It causes increased uptake of amino acids by the target cells, which use them for production of proteins. It inhibits formation of fat and accelerates the breakdown of any fat stores in the body. Overall, it can be seen that growth hormone stimulates anabolic metabolism (anabolism = building up of tissues; catabolism = metabolic breakdown or utilisation of tissues, as in starvation).

A variety of factors cause release of growth hormone, and at the present time the exact mechanism of control is not clear. Lack or excess of GH is one reason for an individual becoming a dwarf or giant, compared with others of the species or breed.

(4) **Gonadotropins**
These hormones stimulate the development of the gonads, and there are two hormones to be considered.

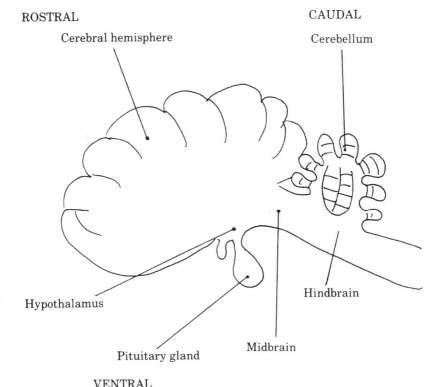

ROSTRAL   CAUDAL

Cerebral hemisphere   Cerebellum

Hypothalamus   Hindbrain

Pituitary gland   Midbrain

VENTRAL

Figure 9-2. The pituitary gland.

117

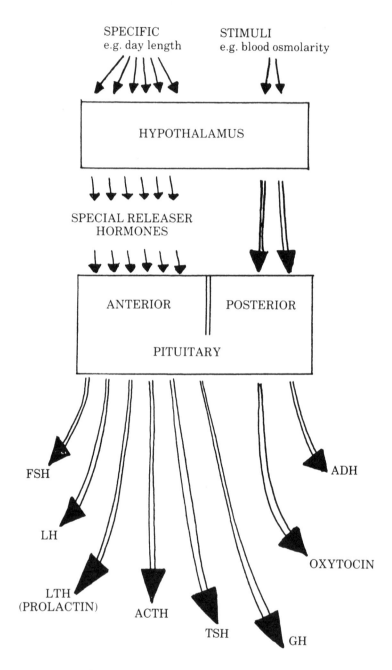

Figure 9-3. Pituitary and hypothalamus.

118

(a) **Follicle Stimulating Hormone** (FSH)
In the female this acts on the ovary to cause the growth and subsequent maturation of ovarian follicles which contain the ova (Chapter 13). In the male, the same hormone stimulates growth of the seminiferous tubules (the site of sperm production within the testes), and has an influence on the actual process of sperm production.

(b) **Luteinizing Hormone** (LH)
LH is responsible for causing the release of the mature ova from the ovarian follicle, and the formation of the corpus luteum within the ovary. In some species, e.g. cats, it is known that LH is only released following vaginal stimulation at the time of mating. The cells of the follicle produce the female sex hormones (oestrogens) and the corpus luteum is an important source of progesterone (though not the only one, according to species). Progesterone is one of the hormones contributing to the maintenance of pregnancy (Chapter 13).

In the male, LH causes the interstitial cells of the testis to produce male sex hormones, which are collectively called androgens, the most important of which is testosterone. 'Male' and 'female' hormones are not exclusive to their sex; hormones of the opposite sex are found but in much smaller concentrations. This varies with the individual and the species. Some of these hormones come from the adrenal cortex (see below).

(5) **Prolactin**
The prime site of action of prolactin is the mammary glands where it causes development of mammary tissue and stimulates lactation. The secretion of prolactin rises during pregnancy, and levels remain high during lactation. The effect of prolactin on cells is similar to that of growth hormone, stimulating amino acid uptake and protein synthesis.

The anterior pituitary is not autonomous: it is controlled by the hypothalamus. In fact the hypothalamus does this by producing special local hormones which travel via a direct portal blood system to the anterior pituitary, causing it to release one or other of its hormones. The relationship between the hypothalamus and the posterior pituitary is even closer: it is a down-growth from the hypothalamus and serves to store and release hormones which are actually made within that very important area of the brain. We should not be surprised that brain cells can produce hormones; all nerve cells ultimately work by producing very special chemicals such as acetyl choline or noradrenaline (Chapter 10). In fact adrenaline, which is very similar, is a hormone (see below). The real difference is that the chemicals from nerves usually have very specific *local* actions, e.g. on an adjacent nerve, muscle or gland cell. For this reason they are called transmitters – they transmit the message from the nerve (Chapter 10).

The hormones released from the **posterior pituitary** are:

(1) **Vasopressin** (Chapter 7)
This is also called antidiuretic hormone (ADH), it is released in response to an increase in the osmolarity of blood. This is detected by special receptors in the hypothalamus.

119

Vasopressin's target organ is the kidney, where it causes resorption of water from the collecting tubules. A failure to release vasopressin leads to production of an excessive amount of very dilute urine; this is the condition of diabetes insipidus.

(2) Oxytocin

This hormone is involved in both parturition (birth – Chapter 13) and lactation.

At parturition distension of the vagina by the emerging foetus causes a reflex secretion of oxytocin by the pituitary gland. Oxytocin acts on the muscles of the uterine wall (which at this stage are very sensitive to it) causing muscle contraction with subsequent expulsion of the foetus. Oxytocin is also released in response to the young pup or kitten suckling at the mammary gland. Again, by means of a reflex arc, oxytocin is released and it travels in the blood to the mammary gland where it causes the expulsion of milk.

In both these situations, one observes a reflex arc, in which the sensory (or afferent) section involves the nervous system, and the effector (or efferent) system involves the release of a chemical messenger into the blood. It is a good example to demonstrate the often close association between the nervous and endocrine systems, the two main regulatory systems of the body.

THE THYROID GLAND

The paired thyroid glands are situated in the neck, on either side of the trachea, just caudal to the larynx. They are very close to the carotid artery and jugular vein (Fig. 9-4).

"Thyroxine" is produced by the thyroid glands, and a small amount of iodine is required for its production. In fact the term "thyroxine" encompasses at least two hormones ('T_3' and 'T_4') with very similar chemical structures, both containing iodine; the precise differences need only worry biochemists! Thyroxine is produced in response to TSH acting on the gland, and raised levels of thyroxine will normally inhibit further release of TSH from the pituitary, another good example of a negative feedback control system.

The effects of thyroxine are many, but, in general, the hormone stimulates metabolism in the tissues of the body. Raised levels of thyroxine (seen in hyperthyroidism) lead to increased levels of activity and weight loss (often despite an associated increase in appetite!). Affected animals also have a high pulse rate. In contrast, reduced levels of thyroxine (as in hypothyroidism) result in animals being sluggish and dull; they are unable to tolerate a cold environment and they have muscle weakness. In addition, there is often a loss of hair and thickening of the underlying skin. Although hypothyroidism can be due to inadequate levels of iodine in the diet, this is rarely the cause, since commercial foods contain more than sufficient. Hypothyroidism occurring prior to skeletal maturity leads to reduced rates of growth of bone and muscles; it is, therefore, another possible cause of dwarf stature.

120

CRANIAL

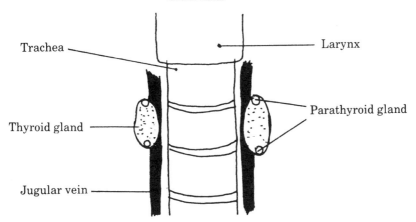

Figure 9-4. Anatomical relationships of thyroid and parathyroid glands.

Calcitonin is a second hormone produced in the thyroid gland. This plays a minor role in maintenance of calcium homeostasis; calcitonin is released in response to raised levels of calcium in the blood and stimulates deposition of calcium in bone, thus reducing plasma calcium back to its normal concentration. Calcitonin is far less important than parathormone (from the parathyroid glands) in maintaining calcium homeostasis; its greatest importance is in growing animals. Calcitonin is produced from a typical minority of cells ('c' cells) which do not produce thyroxine; in fact they do not share the same embryological origin as the more typical thyroid cells.

THE PARATHYROID GLANDS

These are small glands situated next to the thyroid glands. There are usually four parathyroid glands, with one situated at each pole of each thyroid gland (Fig. 9-4). Parathormone (PTH) is produced by these glands, and plays a vital role in maintaining calcium homeostasis, acting to raise the level of calcium in the blood.

A lowering of plasma calcium concentration below a critical "threshold" leads to a rapid disruption of nerve and muscle function; in addition blood clotting will be impaired. The parathyroid glands respond to this fall by releasing parathormone which will raise plasma calcium by:

(a) Reducing calcium loss through urine; PTH stimulates calcium reabsorption in the distal tubule (thus fulfilling a role for calcium similar to that of aldosterone for sodium: Chapter 7).

(b) Increased breakdown of bone, so liberating calcium into the blood.

(c) Increased formation of "metabolically active" vitamin D, which itself stimulates absorption of calcium in the small intestine. As we saw in Chapter 7, active vitamin D is thus another hormone, one of several produced by the kidneys.

121

Once plasma calcium is raised above the "threshold" a process of negative feedback switches off PTH release. This is one of several mechanisms which regulate plasma Ca^{++} (Fig. 9-5) and it is probably the most important.

Overactivity of the parathyroid glands occurs in animals fed on a diet rich in phosphorus and deficient in calcium; an example is an "all meat" diet, without any added cereal. Similarly, overactivity of the parathyroids is encountered in animals with severe renal disease, without sufficient active vitamin D for adequate intestinal absorption of calcium. Prolonged high levels of parathormone lead to extensive resorption of calcium from bones and may lead to such weakening of the bones that they bend or fracture! Occasionally, animals with advanced renal disease lose so much bone mineral that their jaws become bendy ("rubber jaw").

THE ADRENAL GLANDS

The paired adrenal glands lie in the abdomen, just cranial to the kidneys. Each gland is divided into two: a central medulla, and the peripheral cortex. Both regions have endocrine functions but they produce different hormones (Fig. 9-6).

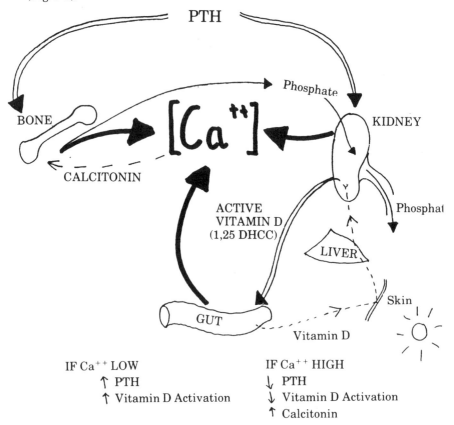

IF Ca^{++} LOW
↑ PTH
↑ Vitamin D Activation

IF Ca^{++} HIGH
↓ PTH
↓ Vitamin D Activation
↑ Calcitonin

Figure 9-5. Regulation of plasma Ca^{++}.

122

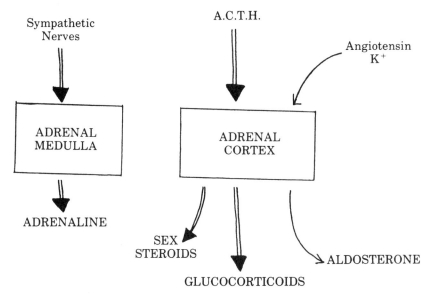

Figure 9-6. Adrenal gland.

The cells of the **adrenal cortex** produce a number of steroid hormones, and the main control of adrenal cortical function is ACTH released by the anterior pituitary gland. The major hormones produced at the adrenal cortex are:

(1) **Cortisol**

This is a "glucocorticoid", and effects a rise in the level of blood glucose as well as stimulating protein breakdown. It inhibits the inflammatory response, hence the use of glucocorticoids as "anti-inflammatory" drugs (corticosteroids) by veterinary surgeons. It also stimulates appetite and enhances water loss at the kidney (by blocking the action of vasopressin). This explains some of the side-effects of long-term steroid therapy in animals, namely a ravenous appetite and increased urine production, with an associated increase in thirst. Raised levels of cortisol act at the pituitary to inhibit ACTH release (negative feedback).

(2) **Aldosterone**

Aldosterone is a "mineralocorticoid", playing a role in maintaining a correct mineral (primarily sodium and potassium) balance in the body. Aldosterone is released in response to raised levels of circulating angiotensin (produced, indirectly, by the kidney) in response to reduced blood flow to the glomerulus. The effect of aldosterone is to increase sodium resorption from the distal tubule of the nephron, also from the colon (hence faeces) and, in us, from sweat. The overall effect is to expand the extracellular fluid volume (negative feedback: Chapter 7).

(3) **Sex Hormones**

Sex hormones, both androgens and oestrogens, are produced from the adrenal cortex; their exact significance is not clear since the gonads produce a plentiful supply.

123

Clinically, there are two important endocrine disorders involving the adrenal cortex. In hyperadrenocorticism (Cushing's disease), clinical signs are due to an excess of circulating cortisol leading to increased thirst, increased urination, the breakdown of muscles and hair loss. By contrast, the effects of reduced activity of the adrenal cortex are attributable to a lack of aldosterone. There is a loss of sodium ions in the urine, and retention of potassium ions. The result is a dramatic collapse of the extracellular fluid volume together with a rise in plasma K^+; this may lead to the death of the animal. This condition of hypoadrenocorticism is called Addison's disease.

The cells of the **adrenal medulla** produce adrenaline and noradrenaline (also called epinephrine and norepinephrine, respectively). Release of these hormones is stimulated by automomic (or visceral) nerves which pass to the adrenal medulla. Both hormones have similar effects and prepare an animal for dangerous or stressful situations (e.g. being threatened by another, perhaps larger, animal); they are thus associated with "fright, fight or flight". The sympathetic nervous system (Chapter 10) has very similar effects, but the hormones last longer. Through their action on the cardiovascular system they raise the heart rate and blood pressure as well as diverting blood away from the visceral organs (e.g. stomach and intestines) towards the skeletal muscles of the body; they are vasoconstrictors for most tissues but in some they increase blood flow. They cause an elevation of the blood glucose level by stimulating breakdown of glycogen in the liver. Hence, the animal is prepared rapidly either to "stand its ground" and fight, or run "like the wind" to escape from the aggressor! You have all experienced the effects of adrenaline during extreme fear, anger or excitement, e.g. becoming pale with terror (skin vasoconstriction). We even speak of "getting the adrenaline going" e.g. athletes before a big event – or students before an exam!

THE GONADS

Both the ovary and the testis are important sites for the production of sex hormones.

Oestrogens are produced in the ovary; they are responsible for causing the development of secondary sexual characteristics, e.g. development of mammary glands. During the early phase of oestrus there are high levels of oestrogen which cause behavioural changes making the female more "attractive" to males, and also more receptive.

The corpus luteum forms in the remains of the ovarian follicle, following ovulation, and it produces progesterone. Progesterone is often referred to as the "hormone of pregnancy", since it is essential for an animal to sustain pregnancy. It acts on the uterus creating conditions which allow the implantation and subsequent development of the embryo. The placenta is an alternative source of progesterone (Chapter 13).

In the male, testosterone is produced by the interstitial cells of the testis. It acts both locally, promoting sperm development in the seminiferous tubules, and at more distant sites within the body where it stimulates the development and maintenance of the accessory sexual glands (e.g. the prostate). Testosterone is responsible for maintaining sexual drive; low levels of testosterone will lead to reduced sexual drive, or a lack of "libido".

Unlike the other endocrine glands, the gonads only become fully active once the animal is mature, i.e. at puberty.

HORMONES

Although we have talked about the great variety of effects of different hormones, they also have a lot in common.

Since hormones are chemical messengers delivered to their target tissues by the blood, the crucial factor is their plasma concentration. Usually this changes through appropriate alterations in the rate of secretion – but it can also change through variations in the rate of breakdown and excretion, e.g. in liver or kidney disease. Hormone concentration in plasma can be measured as an aid to diagnosis. Basically there are two main ways of doing this;

(a) Bio-assay which looks at the effect of the hormone concentration in the sample on a suitable system, and

(b) Competitive binding assays (immuno-assays). These measure the concentration of the hormone chemically using antibodies which bind to the specific structural characteristics of the hormone.

As regulator substances, hormones are typically involved in negative feedback loops which prevent oversecretion or reduce secretion once the appropriate effect has been achieved. We have already seen that these can be multiple loops, for example, glucocorticoid secretion can be suppressed either via its effects on blood glucose or simply by suppressing the release of ACTH from the anterior pituitary. The existence of feedback loops is important in treatment; supplying the hormone as a drug will also tend to damp down the animal's own production of the hormone, and this may recover only slowly when the drug stops, e.g. extended corticosteroid treatment. Sometimes we encounter positive feedback loops which accelerate secretion, e.g. oestrogens reinforce the release of gonadotropins, which in turn accelerate follicular ripening and oestrogen production.

Hormones are very potent chemicals and many are readily absorbed through the skin or the intestine; when used for treatment they should be handled with care. Some hormones are deliberatey administered via skin patches.

You might wonder why all hormones do not affect all tissues and why, instead, most hormones have very specific targets. The main reason is that the cells need specific receptors to allow the hormone to attach. The hormone does not necessarily enter the cell at all; often the binding to the receptor releases a "second chemical messenger" which actually enters the cells and triggers the effects which we attribute to the hormone. So although most cells are exposed to most hormones, the only ones affected are those with the correct receptors (or switches) and with the ability to produce the specific response. The detailed manner of action of hormones is complicated and

125

outside the needs of your course but it relates mainly to the chemical nature of the hormone; most hormones are proteins (e.g. GH), peptides (e.g. ADH), steroids (e.g. oestrogen) or fatty acids (e.g. prostaglandins).

Prostaglandins are an unusual group of hormones, being produced in a variety of tissues and having a variety of effects including involvement in fever (Chapter 4), inflammation, regulation of blood flow and reproduction. An important group of drugs oppose some of their effects, notably on inflammation and fever. Like corticosteroids these drugs are thus anti-inflammatory and are known as 'non-steroidal anti-inflammatories' (NSAI's). Not surprisingly, they also tend to reduce fever and the prototype was Aspirin, still in use alongside phenylbutazone, ibuprofen, flunixin, etc.

Increasingly we find that drugs act by stimulating or blocking receptors whose natural stimulus would be a hormone. In some cases this knowledge is very new, even though the drugs are very old. For example, opiates (e.g. morphine, codeine, fentanyl, etorphine – as in 'Immobilon') utilise the receptors for natural pain-killers known as endorphins. Similarly cardiac glycosides (digitalis) utilise the receptors for natural hormones regulating sodium movement out of cells. This should not be as surprising as it seems; potentially the most refined way to alter body function (with a drug) must be to take advantage of the natural control systems, notably hormones.

CHAPTER 10:
THE NERVOUS SYSTEM

There can be little doubt that the nervous system is the most complex of the body's systems. However, this should not prevent one gaining a basic understanding of its anatomy and physiology and using this to understand some of the neurological disorders observed in domestic animals.

The nervous system is the body's major control system, particularly for rapid responses and for 'voluntary' activity. It receives information (from both the internal and external environments), interprets this, and then initiates appropriate actions. On an anatomical basis, the major components of the nervous system are:

1. The central (or processing and interpreting) components: the central nervous system (CNS)

2. The sensory (or afferent) components (afferent = leading *towards* the CNS)

3. The motor (or efferent) components (efferent = leading *away* from the CNS). 'Motor' means driving a tissue to respond, not just causing movement.

However, despite this conventional attempt to categorise the parts of the nervous system, the exact function of many areas remains unclear.

The nervous system may also be divided into somatic and autonomic components. Autonomic fibres serve smooth muscle and glandular structures, i.e. those parts not normally under conscious control, whereas the somatic fibres serve all other structures in the body, especially skeletal muscle.

THE NEURON

The neuron is the basic cell in the nervous system; it is specialised to allow the conduction of nervous impulses along its length. The components of the neuron are (Fig. 10-1):

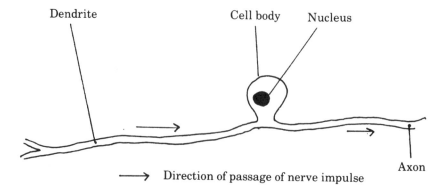

Direction of passage of nerve impulse

Figure 10-1. Structure of a simple neuron.

1. The cell body, which contains the nucleus.
2. Cell processes which lead to and from the cell body.

The cell processes are called nerve fibres, and may be divided into two types:

A. The axon, which carries impulses away from the cell body
B. The dendrite, which carries impulses towards the cell body.

The fundamental property of a nerve cell is that its membrane is electrically charged thanks to active pumping of ions, especially Na^+ and K^+ (Chapter 5). Although this voltage is small, its discharge (depolarisation), transmitted along the length of the nerves, allows them to act as high-speed electrical signalling systems. After the signal passes, the membrane is recharged, using energy (ATP) to restore the Na^+ and K^+ to their resting position.

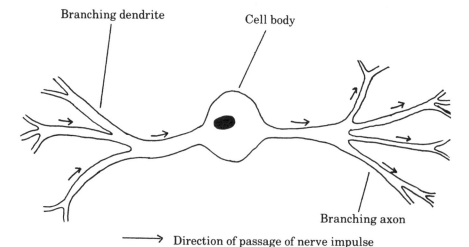

Direction of passage of nerve impulse

Figure 10-2. Structure of a complex neuron.

128

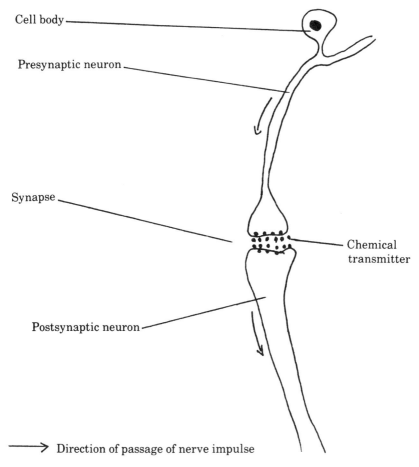

Cell body

Presynaptic neuron

Synapse

Chemical transmitter

Postsynaptic neuron

⟶ Direction of passage of nerve impulse

Figure 10-3. Structure of a synapse.

Both dendrites and axons may be singular or branched structures (Fig. 10-2). Branching of dendrites allows convergence of signals (impulses) from numerous sites towards the cell body, and branching of axons allows divergence of nervous impulses away from the cell body. The nervous system is thus well suited to its function as a communication network.

The junction between two or more neurons is called a synapse, and there is a small gap between the neurons (Fig. 10-3). Electrical impulses cannot pass across this gap, so communication is dependent upon a chemical transmitter. The electrical impulse in the first (or presynaptic) neuron causes release of a transmitter which diffuses across the gap and binds to receptor sites on the membrane of the second (or postsynaptic) neuron. Here it may cause depolarisation of the membrane, leading to generation of a nervous impulse (an excitatory synapse), or may stabilise the membrane, preventing an impulse from occurring (an inhibitory synapse). The junction between a

129

neuron and a muscle cell is very similar; this is called the neuromuscular junction. Several different chemical transmitters have been identified at synapses but the commonest are acetyl choline (often abbreviated to Ach) and noradrenaline. Since one side of the synapse is modified to produce the transmitter, and the other to receive it, synaptic transmission is one-way only. After it has activated the synapse, acetyl choline is rapidly broken down by an enzyme (cholinesterase) so that the single impulse reaching the synapse does not cause an unending stream of impulses in the next neuron. Interference with this enzyme will, however, produce excessive parasympathetic activity (see below), hence the toxicity of 'anticholinesterase' drugs. 'Nuvan' is such a drug which, correctly used, interferes with the nervous system of fleas and lice but, incorrectly used, it may do the same to the dog or cat. Not all transmitters excite the next neuron, there are some which serve to inhibit activity.

Neurons are not the only cell type in the nervous system, but are surrounded by a large number of supporting (or glial) cells. These provide structural support for the very delicate neurons and also provide some nutrients. The supporting cells produce an insulating layer, composed of a fatty material called myelin, which is deposited around many nerve fibres. The myelin sheath increases the rate of electrical conduction along these nerve fibres and is responsible for their white colour. The fact that the nervous system is basically an electrical signalling system is the basis of two types of diagnostic test. The electroencephalogram is a measure of the overall patterns of electrical activity transmitted from the brain and the waveforms show characteristic changes with certain forms of activity (e.g. sleep) or disease (e.g. epilepsy). The integrity of some peripheral nerves can be assessed by using a suitable stimulator and recorder to measure their speed of conduction.

THE REFLEX ARC

The simplest arrangement of neurons is seen in a reflex arc (Fig. 10-4). Stimulation of a sensory receptor in the skin produces an impulse in the afferent or sensory neuron. This passes along the neuron to a synapse (situated in the spinal cord). Release of a transmitter stimulates the effector, or motor neuron. The nervous impulse will cause muscles to contract in response to the initial stimulus. The reflex thus links a sensory stimulus to an automatic response – no 'thought' (i.e. conscious brain activity) is required. For example, if a dog's paw touches a sharp surface, e.g. broken glass, it will immediately withdraw the leg. This is an example of a monosynaptic reflex (there being only one synapse involved in the reflex arc). Because electrical transmission is fast compared with chemical transmission (at each synapse), every synapse introduces a slight delay – hence the very rapid response obtainable from a monosynaptic reflex.

This is somewhat over-simplified since reflex arcs are invariably more complex than this. Returning to the dog treading on a piece of broken glass, then the afferent nerve not only synapses with the efferent neuron, as described, but also synapses with neurons (intermediate or connector neurons) which pass up the spinal cord to the brain. The dog is thus consciously aware of the painful stimulus, and will look around at the affected

130

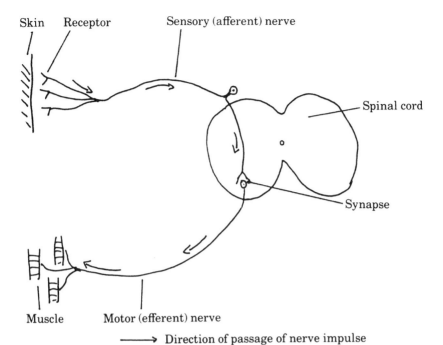

Skin   Receptor   Sensory (afferent) nerve

Spinal cord

Synapse

Muscle   Motor (efferent) nerve

⟶ Direction of passage of nerve impulse

Figure 10-4. Diagram to illustrate a simple reflex arc.

foot. It may initiate other motor actions, including whimpering, and moving its whole body away from the sharp object; these would not be possible with the monosynaptic reflex alone.

The communication between the reflex arc and the brain, via the spinal cord, may also function in the opposite direction. Consider the control of urination: as urine accumulates the bladder wall is distended. Once a critical volume is reached there is contraction of muscles in the bladder wall and urination begins. This is mediated by a local reflex arc. Such a sequence of events is observed in young animals who have poor conscious control over urination. However, the reflex arc may be suppressed by impulses passing from the brain to the spinal cord, and inhibiting the motor neuron. This occurs in the house-trained dog; filling of the bladder does not immediately lead to urination, but instead the dog is aware that urine is accumulating and can consciously inhibit urination until such time that it can go out into the garden. The same is true of ourselves; we can usually inhibit this reflex and only urinate at a convenient (and socially acceptable!) time. We are also aware that other reflex responses vary in their sensitivity or intensity according to our state of mind, e.g. the response to a sudden loud noise, or a needle-prick.

RECEPTORS AND EFFECTORS

The receptors of the nervous system are widespread in the body, and respond to changes in the internal and external environments.

131

The receptors for monitoring the external environment are situated in the skin and mucous membranes (Chapter 2) and are responsive to mechanical, thermal, and painful, or noxious, stimuli. In addition there are receptors of the special senses (taste, vision, etc; Chapter 11). Although the stimulation of pain receptors usually results in the animal feeling pain, the actual perception of the pain occurs in the brain, in response to the incoming signals from the pain receptors. The nervous system also contains a pain-suppressing system which uses endogenous opiates (endorphins) as transmitters. Stimulation of this system is probably the basis of acupuncture.

Receptors monitoring the internal environment lie in internal organs. The term "mechanoreceptors" describes receptors which detect alterations in the mechanical environment. Those lying in the wall of hollow organs detect changes in tension in the wall. In the intestinal wall they play a role in co-ordinating peristalsis. Similar receptors in the wall of the urinary bladder detect filling of the bladder. A second type of mechanoreceptor is called a proprioceptor which responds to alterations in the tension within muscles and tendons. Mechanoreceptors in joints respond to changes in the angle of the joints.

Baroreceptors and chemoreceptors detect alterations in blood pressure and the oxygenation of blood, respectively (Chapter 6).

Efferent or motor neurons run in the body to synapse with muscle fibres or glandular tissue. Efferent neurons of the somatic (or voluntary) nervous system innervate skeletal (or voluntary) muscles. In contrast, smooth (or involuntary) muscle is innervated by neurons of the autonomic nervous system, and is present in the walls of blood vessels, the bronchial walls, in the walls of internal organs, in the iris of the eye (Chapter 11), and in the skin (Chapter 2).

Salivary glands are innervated by efferent neurons of the autonomic nervous system, and nerve impulses can cause secretion of saliva. This may occur as part of a reflex in response to food being placed in the mouth (Chapter 8).

ARRANGEMENT OF THE NERVOUS SYSTEM

Although the structure and function of the basic unit (the neuron) of the nervous system has been discussed in the context of a typical reflex arc, it is necessary to have some understanding of the arrangement and distribution of neurons within the body.

The nervous system can be divided into the central nervous system (CNS), comprising the brain and spinal cord, and the peripheral nervous system (PNS), comprising the cranial nerves and the spinal nerves.

CENTRAL NERVOUS SYSTEM

The brain lies in the cranium, within the skull and is protected by the overlying bones. The spinal cord leaves the cranium through a hole, the foramen magnum (situated on the caudo-ventral surface of the skull) and runs in the vertebral canal. Mechanical protection is provided by the surrounding vertebrae.

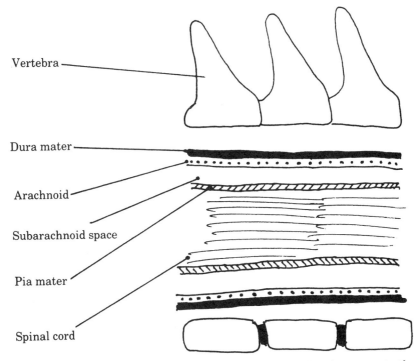

Figure 10-5. Longitudinal section of the vertebral canal to demonstrate the meninges.

The central nervous system is covered by a protective layer of membranes, called the meninges. Inflammation of the membranes is termed meningitis, a condition which may be life-threatening since disease can spread from the meninges to the underlying nervous tissue.

There are three layers of meninges (Fig. 10-5):

1. The **dura mater;** this is the outermost layer, and is a tough fibrous membrane.

2. The **arachnoid;** lies just beneath the dura mater, and is in close contact with it.

3. The **pia mater;** this is the innermost membrane, and covers the nervous tissue of the central nervous system.

Between the arachnoid and the pia mater lies the subarachnoid space which contains a thin, watery fluid called cerebrospinal fluid (CSF). This is also found in the central canal of the spinal cord. CSF serves as a protective fluid jacket around the central nervous system; it also helps maintain a constant environment for the CNS. Cerebrospinal fluid is continuously produced by the brain, and then resorbed into the venous system draining the central nervous system. An excessive amount of fluid (usually resulting from failure of the resorption mechanisms) leads to the condition of hydrocephalus (water on the brain) which is occasionally seen in young puppies and kittens.

133

Myelography is a special radiographic technique which involves the injection, under general anaesthesia, of a radio-opaque dye into the subarachnoid space. The injection is usually made at the junction between the skull and the first cervical vertebra. In the normal animal the dye flows along the subarachnoid space, outlining the spinal cord. In some diseases of the spinal cord, e.g. prolapse of an intervertebral disc or tumour of the spinal cord, there may be obstruction to flow of cerebrospinal fluid at the lesion, and its exact position can be demonstrated by myelography.

The structure of capillaries in the central nervous system differs significantly from the capillaries found elsewhere in the body, since they lack fenestrations, or holes, which allow molecules to pass between the blood and the interstitial space. For molecules to enter the brain they must cross a membrane, hence there is a "blood-brain barrier" which controls the entry and exit of molecules. Molecules which are lipid-soluble, i.e. will dissolve in fat, move across the barrier easily, whereas electrically charged substances, which have a low lipid solubility, will not. The blood-brain barrier thus controls the penetration of drugs into the brain and generally those with a higher lipid solubility pass more easily across the barrier. This is important with regard to the use of general anaesthetics. Pentobarbitone (Sagatal) has a much lower lipid solubility than thiopentone (Intraval); the latter, therefore, passes more rapidly into the brain. The result is a more rapid induction of anaesthesia following injection of thiopentone than with pentobarbitone.

THE BRAIN

The brain is the central control station of the nervous system; the switchboard. It receives sensory information, processes this, and, if appropriate, institutes a response. Although analogies have been drawn between computers and the brain such a comparison belittles the attributes and properties of the brain. It is far more complex than a computer, has hundreds of billions of neurons and is capable of functioning autonomously.

A great deal of our knowledge about brain function comes from studies of animals in which there has been damage to certain areas of the brain. This can lead to varying degrees of loss of function with subsequent alteration in body activities.

Grossly the brain is divisible into three main areas (Fig. 10-6) which are interconnected by millions of nerve fibres.

The hindbrain is the most caudally placed section, and is continuous with the spinal cord. Its major components are the cerebellum and the medulla oblongata. The cerebellum has a ridged surface; it is involved in the control of balance, and the co-ordination of locomotion. Damage to the cerebellum may follow infection of kittens in utero with feline panleukopenia virus; this leads to difficulty in balancing, with an inability to walk correctly and often tilting of the head.

The medulla oblongata controls breathing, blood pressure, heart rate, and other vital internal functions; damage to this area is invariably fatal.

134

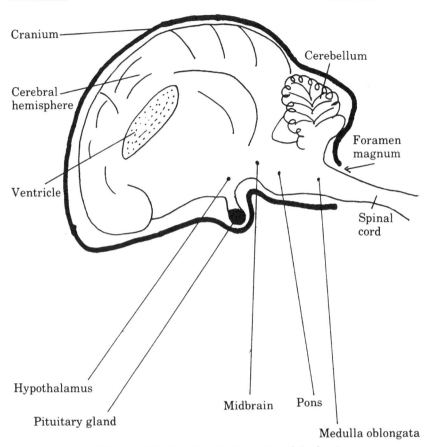

Figure 10-6. Longitudinal section of the brain.

The midbrain is a small area situated deep in the cranium and only seen if the brain is sectioned, since it is overlain by the cerebral hemispheres. The midbrain is responsible for maintenance of the conscious state, so disruption of this region may lead to a state of coma. Neurons in the midbrain are capable of initiating voluntary movement in the body and play an important role in locomotion.

The forebrain is composed of a central section plus two lateral expansions, the cerebral hemispheres. The hemispheres are large structures in the brains of domestic animals, and have an undulating surface, with shallow surface furrows. The hypothalamus lies in the central section of the forebrain and controls the autonomic nervous system. Neurons in the cerebral hemispheres process information relating to smell, taste, vision, hearing, and are sites of learning and personality. They also receive information relating to pain, and play a role in the control of motor function. Thought, memory and awareness

135

are essentially functions of the cerebral hemispheres (cerebral cortex). The object of general anaesthesia is to reversibly block consciousness and perception, including pain perception, without interfering with other functions of the nervous system such as the regulation of breathing and blood pressure. Sleep is different; there is some loss of pain perception but the main effect is a loss of awareness. This is highly selective, unlike general anaesthesia or unconsciousness; the animal or person is readily roused by significant stimuli, e.g. certain voices or other sounds. It is a question of their significance rather than their loudness.

THE SPINAL CORD

This extends from the hindbrain, through the foramen magnum and runs in the vertebral canal. Like the brain it is composed of both nerve fibres and cell bodies. Nerves enter and leave the spinal cord at regular intervals, and pass out from the vertebral canal through an intervertebral foramen. Connector neurons provide cranial and caudal communication within the spinal cord and quite complicated reflexes, e.g. the basic pattern of walking, can be co-ordinated by the spinal cord, rather than the brain. A cross-section of the spinal cord demonstrates (Fig. 10-7):

An outer layer of white matter, composed of myelinated nerve fibres which run to and from the brain (similar to large trunks of cabling used in the National Grid system).

A more central H-shaped area of grey matter composed of cell bodies plus some nerve fibres.

A central canal which contains cerebrospinal fluid and runs the complete length of the spinal cord. In the brain, the central canal leads into the ventricles.

Afferent fibres enter the spinal cord by means of the dorsal root, and the cell bodies of these neurons lie in the dorsal root itself. The axon passes into the spinal cord where it synapses with other neurons. The cell body of the efferent neuron lies in the grey matter, and its axon passes out of the spinal cord in the ventral root. Lateral to the spinal cord, but still within the vertebral canal, the dorsal and ventral roots merge to form a spinal nerve, which passes out through the meninges; from this point it is considered part of the peripheral nervous system.

The spinal cord extends from the foramen magnum to terminate at approximately the last lumbar vertebra, although nerves continue to leave the vertebral canal throughout the sacrum and well into the tail region (caudal vertebrae).

DAMAGE TO THE CENTRAL NERVOUS SYSTEM

If neurons in the central nervous system die they cannot be replaced. Destruction of certain regions of the brain, e.g. medulla oblongata, leads to death due to loss of control of vital body functions. By contrast, destruction of some areas of the cerebral hemispheres may have minimal effect on the animal.

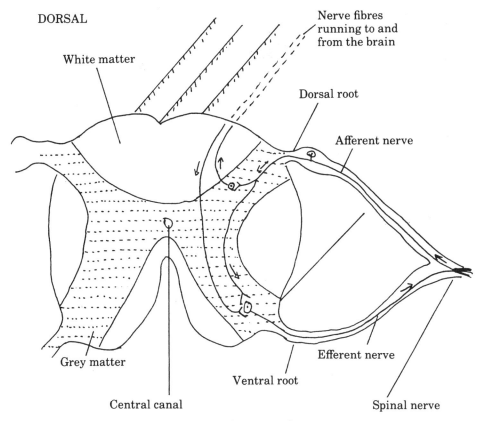

DORSAL

Nerve fibres
running to and
from the brain

White matter

Dorsal root

Afferent nerve

Grey matter

Efferent nerve

Ventral root

Central canal

Spinal nerve

⟶ Direction of passage of nerve impulses

Figure 10-7. Diagrammatic cross-section of the spinal cord
(Meninges omitted for clarity).

In domestic animals it is more common to observe the results of damage to the spinal cord. Complete severance of the cord may follow a fracture of the spine. If this were to occur at the level of the diaphragm there would be loss of voluntary control of muscles caudal to this; the animal will not be able to voluntarily move its hindlegs. Similarly there will be loss of sensation (both conscious and subconscious) from these areas. However, local reflex arcs usually remain intact; if the footpad of the hindpaw is pinched there will be withdrawal of the leg, but the animal will not consciously perceive the pain usually caused by this stimulus. Disruption of spinal cord function can also occur with slowly progressive diseases affecting the neurons. In these cases the clinical signs are gradual in onset, and may specifically affect certain neurons. Dogs with tumours of the spinal cord may initially show slight inco-ordination of the limbs due to loss of neurons involved with proprioception. However, with further growth of the tumour, and destruction of more neurons, voluntary muscle control may be lost leading to paralysis. Damage to the brain or spinal cord does not necessarily interfere with function on the

Table 10-1. THE CRANIAL NERVES

Number	Name	Function
I	OLFACTORY	Smell (SS)
II	OPTIC	Vision (SS)
III	OCULOMOTOR	Motor to extraocular muscles Ps supply to the iris
IV	TROCHLEA	Motor to extraocular muscles
V	TRIGEMINAL	Sensory from the head Motor to major muscles of mastication
VI	ABDUCENS	Motor to extraocular muscles
VII	FACIAL	Motor to muscles of facial expression Ps supply to salivary and lacrimal glands. Taste (SS)
VIII	VESTIBULOCOCHLEAR	Hearing and balance (SS)
IX	GLOSSOPHARYNGEAL	Sensory from mouth and pharynx Motor to pharynx Ps to salivary glands. Taste (SS)
X	VAGUS	Motor and sensory to pharynx and larynx Ps to neck, thorax and abdomen
XI	ACCESSORY	Motor to muscles of cranial neck
XII	HYPOGLOSSAL	Motor to muscles of tongue

KEY: SS = Special sense
Ps = Parasympathetic nerves

same side of the body. Many neural pathways cross to the opposite side of the brain or spinal cord and some functions are associated with only one side of the brain.

THE PERIPHERAL NERVOUS SYSTEM

The peripheral nervous system is composed of the cranial nerves and the spinal nerves.

THE CRANIAL NERVES

There are 12 pairs of cranial nerves which arise directly from the brain, leaving the cranium by a series of small holes in its base and lateral walls. These nerves are responsible for innervating structures of the head, except for the vagus nerve which also innervates structures in the thorax and abdomen. The cranial nerves may have sensory and/or motor functions, and a few are involved in the special senses, e.g. olfactory, optic nerves. Some of the cranial nerves also carry fibres of the autonomic nervous system.

The individual cranial nerves, along with an outline of their function, are listed in Table 10-1.

THE SPINAL NERVES

Spinal nerves contain afferent and efferent somatic fibres, and leave the spinal cord at regular intervals. They innervate voluntary muscles, and receptors in the skin. In the thoracic, lumbar and sacral regions spinal nerves also contain fibres of the autonomic nervous system; these branch off from the spinal nerve close to the vertebral column to innervate visceral structures.

Within the limbs there is not a distinct segmental arrangement of spinal nerves, as seen in the trunk, but instead a system of nerve trunks. These arise from plexuses where spinal nerves enter in a segmental fashion but their fibres undergo regrouping to exit in large trunks; these are given special anatomical names.

In the forelimb the major nerve trunks are the radial, median and ulnar nerves, and between them they supply the majority of somatic structures (both motor and sensory) in this limb. An understanding of the position of the major nerve trunks in the limbs is necessary to avoid causing damage, either at the time of surgery, or when administering an injection. The radial nerve runs caudal to the humerus in the triceps muscle (Fig. 10-8), and passes over the lateral aspect of the distal humerus at the elbow. If the elbow is fractured then the nerve may be damaged, similarly surgical exposure of the humerus for fracture repair must be undertaken carefully to prevent damage to the nerve. Branches of the radial nerve in the forearm run on either side of the cephalic vein. When performing venepuncture, if the needle does not enter the vein correctly it may strike these nerve fibres causing pain and leading to the animal withdrawing its leg (by means of a local reflex).

In the hindleg, the major nerve trunks are the femoral nerve and the sciatic nerve. The sciatic nerve runs in the hamstring muscles caudal to the femur (Fig. 10-9). Intramuscular injections are commonly made in this muscle close to the nerve; it is possible to accidentally inject into the sciatic nerve and damage it.

DISRUPTION OF THE PERIPHERAL NERVOUS SYSTEM

The peripheral nervous system has a poor ability to repair damage so trauma often leads to loss of function. If the radial nerve is severed the animal suffers from radial paralysis. There is loss of function of the extensor muscles (Chapter 12) of the foreleg, there is also loss of sensation from the skin on the cranial surface of the leg. A similar effect can be produced by the temporary interruption of nerve function by infusing local anaesthetic, e.g. lignocaine, around the nerve; this causes the area served by the nerve to become numb. We are probably all aware of this sensation from the use of local anaesthetics

139

in our own mouths at the time of dental treatment. A knowledge of the distribution of the peripheral nerves allows selective inhibition of nerve function using local anaesthetics, so rendering an area of the body free from sensation. This will allow simple surgical procedures to be undertaken (e.g. removal of a wart, suturing a superficial laceration) in the conscious animal. This technique of selective local analgesia is used widely in larger domestic animals, e.g. horse and cow, although it is equally applicable to the dog and cat. Nerves can be anaesthetised close to the area needing to be desensitised or close to their emergence from the spinal cord (epidural and spinal anaesthesia). Permanent denervation may abolish pain but it also makes the animal unaware of damage sustained by the relevant area and is thus potentially dangerous.

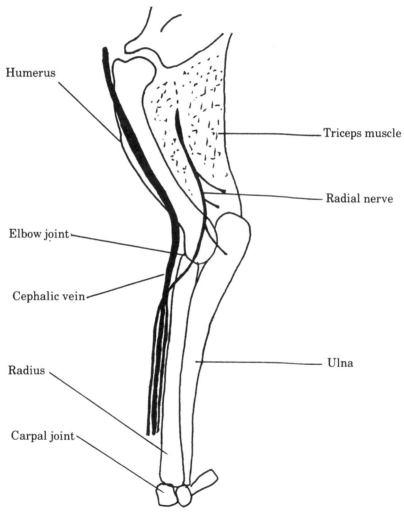

Figure 10-8. Diagram to demonstrate part of the course of the radial nerve.

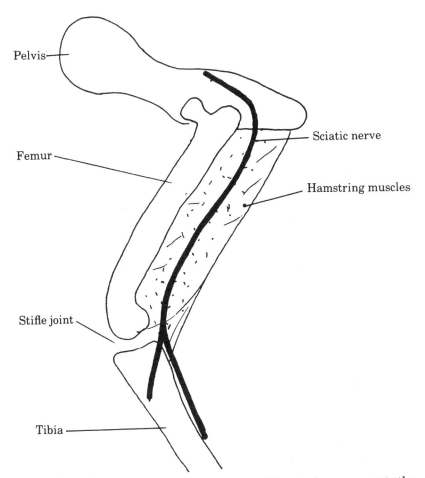

Pelvis

Sciatic nerve

Femur

Hamstring muscles

Stifle joint

Tibia

Figure 10-9. Diagram to demonstrate passage of the sciatic nerve near to the proximal femur.

THE AUTONOMIC NERVOUS SYSTEM

The autonomic nervous system controls many of the internal functions of the body, and is normally self-governing; it usually functions without the conscious knowledge of the animal.

Normally, when referring to the autonomic nervous system, one considers only the efferent or motor components. It is important to realise that there is a sensory component to the autonomic nervous system which detects alterations in the body's internal environment.

In the autonomic nervous system the effector pathway from the spinal cord to the effector organ involves two neurons (unlike the somatic nervous system

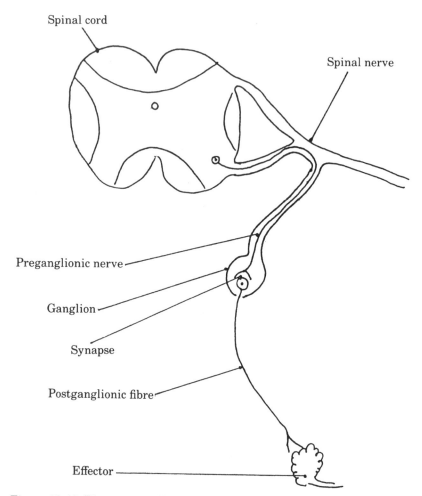

Figure 10-10. Diagram to illustrate the path of efferent neurons in the autonomic nervous system.

which involves only one neuron). The first neuron (or preganglionic fibre) initially runs in a spinal nerve, but then branches from it, to synapse with the second (or postganglionic) neuron (Fig. 10-10). (The term "ganglion" describes a collection of cell bodies lying outside the central nervous system.) Postganglionic fibres pass to the effector tissue.

On the basis of anatomical distribution, function and the chemical transmitter used at the synapse between postganglionic neuron and effector, the autonomic nervous system can be divided into two sections:

1. The Sympathetic Nervous System
Preganglionic fibres originate from the spinal cord in the thoracic and

lumbar regions. Postganglionic fibres are distributed widely to tissues throughout the body, including the head. Structures innervated include smooth muscle in the wall of blood vessels, in the gastrointestinal and urinary tracts and in the iris of the eye. Fibres also innervate the salivary and lacrimal glands.

At the synapse between postganglionic fibre and effector organ, the chemical transmitter is usually noradrenaline. Its effect can be blocked by acepromazine, a drug used widely as a premedicant.

2. The Parasympathetic Nervous System

Preganglionic fibres of the parasympathetic nervous system are present in four of the cranial nerves (Table 10-1), and in the sacral nerves. Fibres running in the cranial nerves innervate structures in the head (lacrimal and salivary glands, the iris); in addition, fibres in the vagus nerve run to the thorax (to innervate the heart and bronchi) and to the abdomen (to innervate structures in the gastrointestinal tract, down to the level of the colon). Parasympathetic fibres arising from the sacral outflow pass in the pelvic nerves to innervate muscle of the bladder, and erectile tissue of the genitalia.

Acetylcholine is the chemical transmitter released by the postganglionic fibres; its effect is blocked by atropine, a drug often used as a premedicant. One of the beneficial actions of atropine is to reduce salivation by interfering with their cholinergic (acetylcholine-dependent) stimulation. It also widens the pupils because they are normally constricted by parasympathetic activity and dilated by sympathetic activity ("wide-eyed with fear").

Stimulation of the sympathetic nervous system produces a state of alertness in the body, with redirection of blood away from skin and gut towards the skeletal muscle, reduction in secretion by exocrine glands, a raising of the heart rate and elevation of blood pressure. This is the same response as occurs with release of noradrenaline and adrenaline from the adrenal medulla (Chapter 9), and is called the "fight or flight" response. In contrast, stimulation of the parasympathetic nervous system causes a slowing of the heart, with increased activity of the gut, and increased secretion by the lacrimal and salivary glands. It is important to realise that the functioning of the two sections of the autonomic nervous system is not mutually exclusive. They usually function together in the normal animal, with the final effect being dependent upon the balance between the two systems. This is demonstrated when drugs block the action of either system. Injecting atropine into a healthy dog will lead to a rise in the heart rate and reduction in salivation (the oral mucous membranes will feel dry). These changes are due to atropine inhibiting the effects of the parasympathetic nervous system. By contrast, injection of a drug which blocks the sympathetic nervous system, e.g. acepromazine, will cause the heart to slow, and blood pressure to fall, due to reduction of the normal sympathetic activity in the body (Chapter 6).

CHAPTER 11:
THE SPECIAL SENSES

The special senses are taste, smell, vision, hearing and balance, all of which are detected by receptors in the head. Some of the receptors are located in special sensory organs, e.g. the eye for vision, whereas others are distributed more widely, e.g. taste receptors in the mouth. All the special senses use cranial nerves (Chapter 10) to relay information to the brain.

THE EYE

The eye is the organ of vision. It is positioned in the orbit, a bony socket which lies just rostral to the cranium and lateral to the nasal cavity and frontal sinus. The position of the eyes in the skull differs between animals and is influenced by their natural habitat. In the dog and cat, which were originally predatory animals, the eyes are positioned well forward in the skull, resulting in a large field of binocular vision. This allows them to gauge distances accurately. By comparison, in grazing animals, e.g. the horse and cow, the eyes are more laterally placed allowing a greater total field of vision, but with a small field of binocular vision. This allows animals to detect approaching danger, e.g. predators, over a wide area.

The eye is a delicate structure, and is protected by the bones of the orbit. The eyelids (palpebrae) are two mobile folds of tissue which cover the front surface of the eye. They contain skeletal muscle and are covered by skin on their outer surface and by a mucous membrane, the conjunctiva, on their inner surface. The eyelids join each other at the lateral and medial canthi (angles) (Fig. 11-1). Hairs (eyelashes) are present in the free edge of the eyelid, and more are present in the upper, or dorsal, lid than the lower, or ventral, lid. Normally the eyelashes grow away from the eye's surface. However, in the condition of distichiasis some of the hairs grow towards, and into, the front surface of the eye, causing inflammation and ulceration.

In most animals (but not man) there is an extra, or third, eyelid called the nictitating membrane. It lies at the medial canthus and is usually white in

145

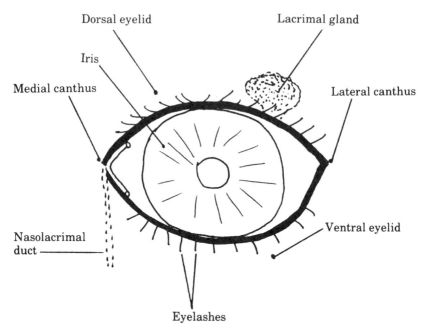

Dorsal eyelid

Lacrimal gland

Iris

Medial canthus

Lateral canthus

Nasolacrimal
duct

Ventral eyelid

Eyelashes

Figure 11-1. The eyelids and lacrimal apparatus.

colour. It contains a small plate of cartilage which is covered by conjunctiva. The eye supports the nictitating membrane in its normal position. When the eye is retracted within the orbit the nictitating membrane is pushed across to cover part of the front surface of the eye. In a dehydrated or emaciated animal the eye sinks in the orbit causing the nictitating membrane to protrude from the medial canthus and become clearly visible when the eyelids are open.

The conjunctiva is a transparent mucous membrane covering the inner surface of the eyelids, the nictitating membrane and part of the sclera of the eye.

Both the cornea and the conjunctiva are kept moist by tears produced by the lacrimal gland which lies under the dorsal eyelid (Fig. 11-1). Production of tears is controlled by the autonomic nervous system: the parasympathetic nerves stimulate tear secretion, whereas the sympathetic nerves inhibit it. Tears drain via the nasolacrimal duct, which runs from the medial canthus to the nasal cavity.

Damage to the lacrimal gland often results in failure of tear production. This leads to the condition of keratoconjunctivitis sicca, or "dry eye", in which the conjunctiva and cornea become inflamed and infected due to the absence of tears. Vision is impaired because of increased opacity of these structures. By contrast, there may be a failure of tear drainage due to obstruction of the nasolacrimal duct. Tears will flow out over the eyelids onto the surface of the cheek causing a characteristic discolouration of the hair.

146

EXTERNAL STRUCTURE OF THE EYE

The outer layer of the eye is made up of the sclera (or "white" of the eye) which is composed of opaque fibrous tissue and is continuous with the transparent cornea at the front of the eye. The junction between the cornea and the sclera is called the limbus (Fig. 11-2). The sclera acts as the external skeleton of the eye, helping to maintain the eye's shape and providing an insertion for the extraocular muscles which control movement of the eye in the bony orbit. In addition, the sclera acts as a supporting framework for the internal structures of the eye. The cornea allows light to enter, and leave, the eye; it also plays an important role in the "coarse" focussing of light due to its refractile properties.

Inflammation of the cornea is called keratitis; it is a painful condition and causes opacification of the cornea due to the accumulation of water and

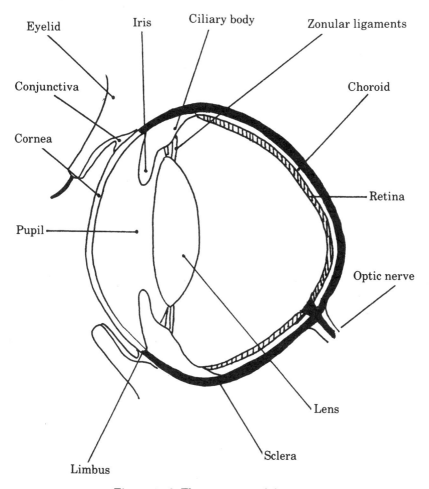

Figure 11-2. The structure of the eye.

147

inflammatory fluid in it. The result is a reduction in the amount of light which can enter the eye and clouding or distortion of the image.

INTERNAL STRUCTURE OF THE EYE

Internally, the eye is divided, by the lens, into the anterior (or front) segment, and the posterior (or back) segment. The anterior chamber contains a watery fluid, called aqueous humour, whereas the posterior chamber contains a thicker, more viscous fluid, the vitreous humour.

The iris is a circular structure situated in the anterior chamber of the eye. It is extremely vascular and contains bands of smooth muscle. The iris is the only internal structure normally seen when examining the eye without the aid of an ophthalmoscope. The iris has an central hole, the pupil, and around its periphery the iris is attached to the ciliary body (Fig. 11-2). Contraction and relaxation of smooth muscle in the iris alters the size of the pupil and controls the amount of light passing to the lens.

Behind the iris is the lens; this is a solid, biconvex structure which is transparent. It is attached to the ciliary body by the zonular ligaments. The lens is normally elastic, and its shape (and consequently its optical properties) is altered by contraction and relaxation of the smooth muscle in the ciliary body. The term "accommodation" describes this alteration in the optical properties of the lens by changes in its shape. The lens is responsible for the "fine" focussing of light onto the retina. The opacity of the lens increases with age in the dog; this is a normal senile change, and does not interfere with vision. This contrasts with cataracts which are abnormal opacities in the lens which interfere with vision by disrupting the passage of light through the lens. Cataracts may be congenital (present at birth). They may also occur in conjunction with other ocular diseases, and occasionally they form in animals with generalised disease, e.g. diabetes mellitus. In certain breeds of dog the development of cataracts has a hereditary basis. If the lens is removed the dog still forms an image without the lens, using the cornea for focussing. Sometimes the lens slips from its normal position, either forwards or backwards (anterior or posterior "luxation").

The retina comprises several layers of specialised nerve receptors which are sensitive to light. The retina lies on the inner surface of the eye, and is supported by an underlying vascular layer called the choroid. Part of the choroid, called the tapetum lucidum, contains pigment which reflects light. The presence of this pigment causes the eyes of dogs and cats to "shine" when observed with a bright light, for example when seen in the beam of car headlights: the original "cats' eyes"! More important, it increases the animal's chances of detecting even dimly lit objects (since the light passes through the retina twice).

The nerve receptors in the retina are responsive to light and are called photoreceptors. Two types are recognised:

Rods, which simply respond to light regardless of colour and function well under low light intensities. They are situated peripherally in the retina and provide the basis of 'night vision'. The distribution of rods in the periphery of

148

the retina explains why animals (including ourselves) see more clearly in the dark if they do not look directly at an object, but instead observe it from an angle.

Cones, which respond to coloured light and function most efficiently under high light intensities. These are positioned more centrally in the retina. In humans there are three different types and, since they are the basis of colour vision, defects give rise to different forms of colour blindness.

Afferent nerve fibres leading from the photoreceptors run on the surface of the retina and leave the eye at the optic disc. When the retina is examined with an ophthalmoscope the optic disc is clearly seen as a circular white structure which has small blood vessels running over it. The optic nerve passes from the optic disc through the back of the eye, and runs through a small hole in the cranium to enter the brain. Nerve fibres run to the cerebral hemispheres where the impulses are interpreted and a visual image is perceived.

OCULAR REFLEXES

(1) **Menace Reflex**
If an object is waved menacingly in front of an animal's eye, without touching the cornea, there is a reflex closure of the eyelids. The reflex arc involves the optic nerve (afferent path) and the facial nerve (efferent path) running to the muscles of the eyelids. Loss of any of the components of this arc, for example if the animal becomes blind, results in loss of this reflex.

(2) **Pupillary Reflex**
When a dog is placed in a dimly-lit room the pupils dilate. If a bright light is then shone into one eye there is an immediate constriction of both pupils, reducing the amount of light passing to the retina. The size of the pupil is controlled by the autonomic nervous system; stimulation of sympathetic nerves causes the pupil to dilate, whereas stimulation of parasympathetic nerves produces constriction of the pupil. The effects of the parasympathetic nerves are blocked by atropine which causes the pupil to dilate. Indeed atropine was once known as 'belladonna' (beautiful woman) because it was used as a 'cosmetic' to make the eyes look wider and darker.

AQUEOUS HUMOUR

Aqueous humour is the watery fluid found in the anterior segment of the eye. It helps supply nutrients to the lens and, because of its refractory properties, helps to focus light. Aqueous humour is continually produced by cells of the ciliary body, and circulates around the anterior chamber. It is resorbed by special cells lying at the junction of the iris and cornea. For various reasons, the resorption of aqueous humour may be interrupted, causing an increase in the amount of fluid present. The result is an elevation of the internal, or intraocular, pressure, causing the eye to bulge. This is the condition of glaucoma and it not only threatens the animal's vision but it is exceedingly painful.

149

THE EAR

The ear serves the special senses of hearing and balance. An understanding of normal structure and function is important since the ear is a common site of disease.

The ear may be divided into three parts.

THE EXTERNAL EAR

This is composed of the pinna (earflap) and the ear canal (Fig. 11-3). The size and shape of the pinna varies considerably between breeds; one needs only to compare the pinna of a German Shepherd Dog with that of a Cocker Spaniel to be aware of this. The pinna is composed of skin and the underlying auricular cartilage. Movement of the pinna is controlled by voluntary muscles. The pinna collects sound waves and directs them into the ear canal; movement of the pinnae puts them in the best position to collect sound from a particular direction. Blood vessels run in the pinna, between the skin and auricular cartilage. Trauma to the pinna may cause the vessels to rupture, with blood accumulating between the cartilage and skin; this is called an aural haematoma.

The ear canal, or auditory meatus, is lined by a layer of modified skin which contains modified sebaceous glands. These are responsible for producing cerumen (ear wax). Support for the external ear is provided by underlying tubular cartilages. There are two sections of the ear canal, the vertical canal and horizontal canal which join at a right-angled bend (Fig. 11-3). The ear canal conducts sound down to the tympanic membrane, which lies at its medial limit. This is a translucent structure, separating the outer ear from the middle ear. In a normal animal, the tympanic membrane can usually be seen when examining the external ear with an auroscope.

Otitis externa describes the condition of inflammation of the external ear. This is very common in both dogs and cats and presenting clinical signs are pain and irritation at the ear with frequent headshaking.

THE MIDDLE EAR

The middle ear lies in the tympanic cavity (Fig. 11-3). It is a bony structure lying on the ventral surface of the skull, close to the articulation of the skull with the lower jaw. The lateral boundary of the middle ear is the tympanic membrane.

The tympanic cavity contains air plus three small bones, the auditory ossicles. Vibrations of the tympanic membrane are transmitted by these bones to the vestibular window which is the junction between the middle and inner ears. There is a communication between the middle ear and the pharynx via the auditory tube (Eustachian tube). The auditory tube opens when an animal swallows and allows equalisation of air pressure on either side of the tympanic membrane. This explains why repeated swallowing can relieve the sensation of "ear popping" often experienced when travelling in an aeroplane as it comes to land. The auditory tube may, however, allow infection to pass from the pharynx up into the middle ear. Inflammation of the middle ear is called otitis media, and may also follow from otitis externa, due to spread of infection through the tympanic membrane.

150

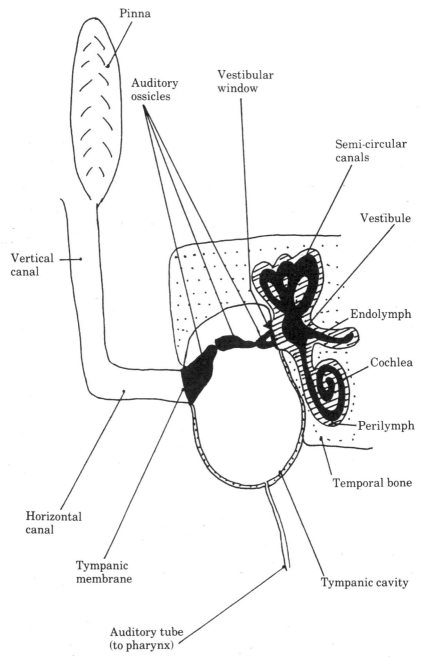

Figure 11-3. The structure of the ear.

151

THE INNER EAR

The inner ear is a very delicate structure situated in a protected site deep within the temporal bone (Fig. 11-3). It is the area where sound vibrations are converted into nervous impulses. In addition, part of the inner ear is involved in maintaining balance. The inner ear comprises a closed system of delicate tubes, called the membranous labyrinth, which contains a fluid, endolymph. The membranous labyrinth is itself bathed in a separate fluid, perilymph, as it sits within the temporal bone.

The major components of the membranous labyrinth are:

(1) **The Vestibule;** a central, sac-like structure from which arise the semi-circular canals and the cochlea.

(2) **The Semi-Circular Canals;** three loop-shaped structures lying at right-angles to each other. Receptors in the wall of the canals respond to movements of endolymph produced by movement of the head. Afferent nerve fibres pass in the vestibulocochlear nerve to the cerebellum. They transmit information on the angle of the head and changes in its position, e.g. rotation. This is used by the cerebellum of the brain to maintain balance. The extreme example of this ability is the falling cat which, provided there is sufficient height (time), always lands on its four feet.

(3) **The Cochlea;** a spiral-shaped structure. It is the area responsible for coverting sound waves into nerve impulses. Vibration of the vestibular window by the auditory ossicles causes wave formation in the perilymph, which is transmitted to the endolymph. This stimulates special receptor cells lying in the wall of the cochlea. Afferent nerve impulses pass in the vestibulocochlear nerve to the cerebral cortex.

The close physical association between the semicircular canals and the cochlea explains why inflammation of the inner ear (otitis interna) may cause deafness and disorders of balance. In fact, of these two senses, disruption of balance is often more apparent clinically since it causes tilting of the head and interferes with locomotion, often causing circling. In comparison, deafness is usually difficult to demonstrate in domestic animals, especially if it affects only one ear.

TASTE

The sense of taste (gustation) involves the response to chemical stimuli in solution, usually associated with the ingestion of food. The receptors are taste cells contained in taste buds which lie in the mucous membrane of the oral cavity (including the tongue), the pharynx, even the larynx. The tongue has several types of papillae on its surface; some, but not all, bear taste buds.

Afferent nerve impulses pass in the glossopharyngeal and facial nerves to the cerebral cortex, where the sense of taste is perceived. Usually stimulation of taste buds lead to salivation and increased activity in the gastrointestinal tract, however, stimulation by noxious chemical stimuli may trigger the vomiting reflex.

SMELL

The sense of smell, or olfaction, is closely linked with that of taste, and is highly developed in both the dog and cat. Smell is important for the selection of food and for the detection of pheromones (Chapter 2). The receptors for smell are located in the mucous membrane of the nasal cavity, and respond to volatile chemicals present in inspired air. Sniffing, by making the airflow more turbulent, helps to divert it towards the areas of the nasal cavities which have most of the olfactory receptors. Afferent nerve fibres run directly from the nasal cavity to the brain by the olfactory nerve. The olfactory mucous membrane can also receive volatile stimuli from the mouth; these gain access via the posterior nares. As a result, much of what we normally think of as taste is actually smell. This becomes obvious when we lose our sense of smell, e.g. during an upper respiratory tract infection; our sense of 'taste' is also badly affected.

BEHAVIOURAL IMPORTANCE OF CHEMICAL SENSES

As in almost all physiology textbooks, this chapter contains less on taste and smell (chemical senses) than vision and hearing. That reflects the fact that more is known about the way in which the eye and ear function – much more than we have recounted here. But that does not necessarily mean that they are more **important** to **animals**. Rather, it results from the fact that blindness and deafness are so important to humans and have provided the drive for so much research. But we are primates and, among the mammals, primates are unusual in having such a highly sophisticated dependence on vision and a relatively poor sense of smell. Our own olfactory acuity, for example, is almost rudimentary compared with that of a dog. In fact dogs can detect chemicals with a precision which, even today, matches the finest analytical equipment. Which is why, in an increasing variety of circumstances, we depend on sniffer dogs to track down people, explosives, drugs, etc.

The dog lives in a world of smells whose variety and excitement we cannot begin to 'visualise' and most mammals are highly dependent on olfaction for their feeding, social, sexual, maternal, territorial, pathfinding, pursuit and avoidance behaviour. Often these involve highly specific chemicals secreted from particular glands (which vary with the species). These chemicals (pheromones) function between animals in the way that hormones function between different organs in the body. In particular, they produce very precise responses in other animals of the same species. Thus the alarmed skunk does not produce a pheromone (it affects various species) but the oestrous bitch (or ewe, or sow, or cow, or mare, or cat) certainly does.

It is, therefore, no surprise that blind dogs manage very well, especially in familiar surroundings; so far as we can guess, they still have their richest source of information and sensory experience – their sense of smell. Olfaction is also important in cats but of course they are more dependent on vision than dogs both for their acrobatics and, in the wild, for their hunting. Perhaps the extreme example of olfactory acuity is in mice, which can recognise others of the same strain with regard to the genes dictating organ transplant compatibility – tissue typing by smell!

153

CHAPTER 12:
THE MUSCULOSKELETAL SYSTEM

The musculoskeletal system comprises the bones of the skeleton, the muscles which attach to them and the nerves and blood vessels required for these tissues to function. Some areas of the musculoskeletal system have already been covered in Chapter 10 when discussing the sensory receptors along with the afferent and efferent nerves.

It is convenient to divide the musculoskeletal system into the skeletal and muscular systems, and consider each separately, but, at the same time, remembering that they function together very closely in the living animal. In addition, although the importance of skeletal muscle is both obvious and visible, there are two other equally important types of muscle; smooth (visceral) and cardiac.

THE SKELETAL SYSTEM

The skeleton is made up of over 200 bones, arranged in an orderly fashion and providing support and protection for the body. Each bone is made up of several tissues, including blood vessels, fibrous tissue, cartilage and bone tissue itself. Bone is a hard tissue which provides the strength of the skeleton. The intercellular matrix of bone is composed of collagen with calcium phosphate deposited in it. The organic matrix of bone is elastic rather than rigid and if there is abnormal loss of bone mineral (mainly clacium and phosphate) bones can become soft and bendy. The strength of healthy bone, like that of reinforced concrete, results from the combined effect of the hard mineral and the flexible organic matrix (like the reinforcing rods). On its own, the mineral is too brittle, as in senile bone. The high calcium content of bone is responsible for its radio-opacity, and bone is clearly seen on radiographs as white areas (since x-rays **blacken** the film tissues which block them appear white). An important fact frequently overlooked is that bone is a living tissue; it contains cells (osteocytes) and has a blood supply; fractured bones often bleed profusely. In many cases our first encounter with bones is as part of a prepared skeleton in which all the surrounding soft tissues, i.e. muscles, tendons, ligaments and blood vessels, have been removed. In many respects this

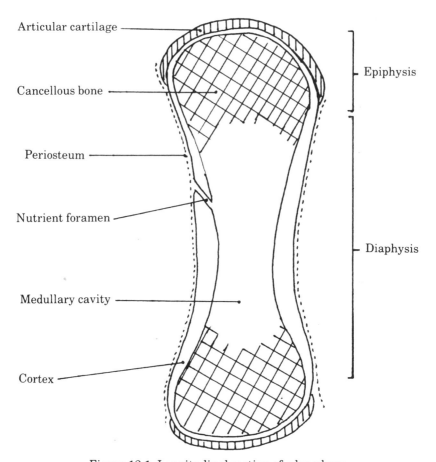

Articular cartilage

Cancellous bone

Periosteum

Nutrient foramen

Medullary cavity

Cortex

Epiphysis

Diaphysis

Figure 12-1. Longitudinal section of a long bone.

provides a rather simplified view of the nature of bone tissue and of the structure and relationship of the bones of the skeleton.

The prime function of the skeletal system is to provide support and protection for the body's internal organs. It also acts as a site for the attachment of muscles which play a role both in locomotion and in the protection of internal organs (e.g. the abdominal wall; Chapter 8). Limb bones are essentially levers operated by the muscles whose tendons attach to them: much of the surface texture and the shape of bones is adapted for these attachments. Bone acts as a reservoir for calcium, which is required for the maintenance of nerve and muscle function. Females often need to draw on this store during pregnancy and lactation. Finally, certain areas of bone contain bone marrow tissue which is responsible for the production of blood cells.

BONE STRUCTURE

The structure of a bone may be studied by sectioning a long bone, for example the femur, or thigh bone (Fig. 12-1). The outer layer of solid or compact bone is

156

called the cortex. It is thickest at the shaft, or diaphysis, of the bone, and thinnest at the ends, or epiphyses. Close examination of compact bone shows that the matrix is laid down in layers (or lamellae) which are closely apposed to each other (similar in some respects to the layers of an onion). The outer surface of the cortex is normally smooth, except at the sites of attachment of muscles or tendons where it may be either raised or depressed. Within the epiphyses, there is predominantly cancellous or spongy bone, in which the matrix is laid down as trabeculae, or struts, in a three-dimensional interlacing pattern, with distinct spaces between them. In the centre of the shaft is the medullary cavity which contains bone marrow. In young animals this contains red marrow which produces red and white blood cells. With ageing this is partially replaced by yellow marrow which contains predominantly fat.

A feature of bone is its ability to repair defects or fractures by producing new bone tissue, rather than forming a scar of fibrous tissue, as occurs in most of the other organs of the body. Moreover, because it is a living tissue, it can 're-model' according to demand. Thus even a misaligned fracture will improve its shape as the limb returns to use, though it will not become normal. Prolonged recumbency causes a loss of bone mass – a result of disuse.

The outer surface of the bone is covered by a fibrous membrane, the periosteum. This is not only the limiting outer membrane of the bone, but it also provides blood to the bone and contains cells which can produce new bone tissue. This is illustrated by the periosteum helping to form the bridging callus at a healing fracture. The periosteum is also very sensitive to pain – a kick on the shins is so painful because there is very little natural padding in humans between the skin and the periosteum at this site. At the epiphyses, the periosteum is continuous with a layer of articular, or hyaline cartilage, which acts as the articular surface of the joint. Cartilage does not normally contain calcium, so is radiolucent, and appears dark on radiographs.

In the shaft of a long bone there is at least one small opening in the cortex, this is the nutrient foramen. The nutrient artery of the bone runs through this into the medullary cavity, where it divides to supply the bone tissue.

As a young animal grows it becomes taller and longer, due primarily to the growth of the bones. Bone growth occurs by two routes. Firstly, new layers of bone can be laid down around the circumference of the shaft, so increasing its diameter. Secondly, longitudinal growth occurs from a layer of cartilage, called the growth plate, which lies between the epiphysis and diaphysis (Fig. 12-2). The cartilage cells divide, expand and then die, to be replaced by bone. This process causes the bone to lengthen. The growth plate is radiolucent (allows x-rays through). At skeletal maturity, the growth plate stops dividing, and is replaced by bone, leading to fusion of the epiphysis and diaphysis. Damage to the growth plate is not uncommon in young dogs, and may lead to shortening of the bone if there is complete cessation of growth. Sometimes, growth is only arrested on one side of the bone, and this leads to an angulation of the bone.

Not all the bones of the body have the structure of a long bone, as described above, belonging instead to the following categories:

157

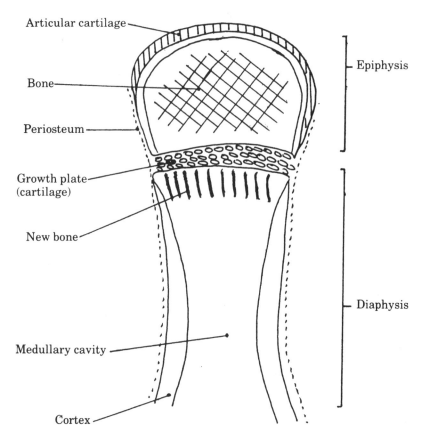

Figure 12-2. Section of a long bone in a young animal to demonstrate the growth plate.

(1) **Flat bones**
As their name suggests, these are flat in shape, and are composed of two layers of cortical bone separated by a small layer of cancellous bone. There is no medullary cavity. Most of the bones of the skull are flat bones.

(2) **Short bones**
These have numerous surfaces and do not contain a medullary cavity. They are composed of an outer layer of cortical bone, with an inner layer of cancellous bone. Short bones are found at the carpus (wrist) and hock (ankle).

(3) **Vertebral bones**
These have an irregular shape and make up the vertebral column. All the bones have a central canal to accommodate the spinal cord (Chapter 10).

(4) **Sesamoid bones**
These are bones formed in tendons (and occasionally ligaments) at points where they alter direction or pass over an underlying bony prominence.

158

The best example is the patella (kneecap) which lies in the tendon of quadriceps femoris muscle. They are not only important to the animal but to anyone looking at an x-ray where, according to the animal's position, they may misleadingly resemble urinary stones or bone fragments.

JOINTS

A joint is formed when two or more bones meet and are joined by elastic, fibrous or cartilaginous tissue, or a combination of the three. Joints are also called articulations (as in lorries).

At a fibrous joint, bones are held rigidly together by fibrous tissue, allowing very little, if any movement. In the skull, fibrous joints hold the bones of the cranium firmly in position, so providing protection for the underlying brain.

Cartilaginous joints have a layer of cartilage between the bones; this allows some movement between the bones. Examples are found at the mandibular symphysis, between the right and left mandibles; and the pelvic symphysis, between the right and left sides of the pelvis. Joints of the pelvis may ease towards parturition.

The greatest amount of movement between bones occurs at synovial joints. Here the bones are separated by a fluid-filled cavity, the synovial cavity. A

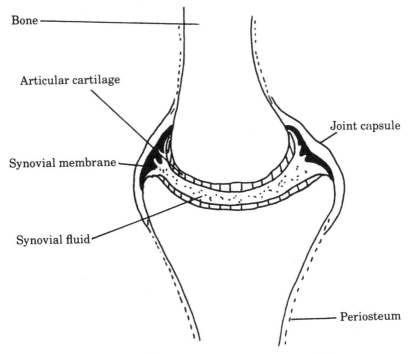

Bone

Articular cartilage

Joint capsule

Synovial membrane

Synovial fluid

Periosteum

Figure 12-3. Diagram of a simple synovial joint.

159

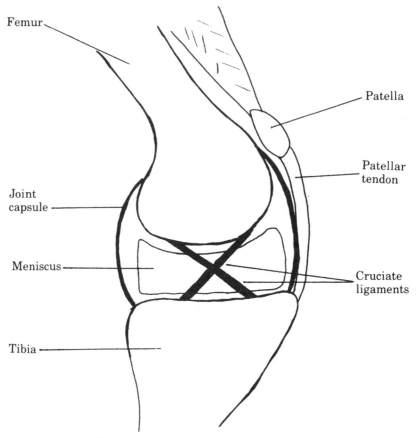

Figure 12-4. Diagram of the stifle joint.

cross-section of a simple synovial joint (Fig. 12-3) shows two layers of articular cartilage separated by synovial fluid. This is normally straw-coloured and slightly viscous. Synovial fluid serves as a joint lubricant; it also helps in the nutrition of the articular cartilage. It is produced by the synovial membrane which lines the synovial cavity. The joint capsule is composed of the synovial membrane plus overlying fibrous tissue; at the edges of the joint the fibrous tissue is continuous with the periosteum of the bones. In some joints, part of the fibrous joint capsule are thickened to form ligaments which provide stability to the joint and restrict movement in certain directions.

Synovial joints may contain intra-articular structures which provide further stability to the joint. At the stifle joint (Fig. 12-4), a complex synovial joint, there are two cruciate ligaments which run from the femur to the tibia, and provide stability to the joint. Rupture of one of these ligaments (usually the cranial or anterior cruciate ligament) is quite common and leads to the joint being unstable, with the animal becoming lame on the affected leg. Intra-articular discs of hyaline cartilage, called menisci (singular: meniscus), are also present in the stifle joint, lying between the femur and tibia. They act as

160

A) Extension and flexion of the elbow joint.

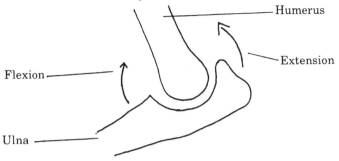

Humerus

Flexion

Extension

Ulna

B) Abduction and Adduction of the forelimb.

Medial

Lateral

Adduction

Abduction

C) Circumduction of the femur.

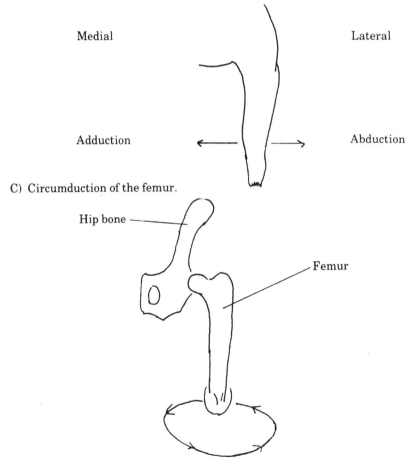

Hip bone

Femur

Figure 12-5. Joint movements.

intra-articular shock absorbers, preventing concussive damage to the articular cartilage. These are the notorious cartilages which trouble sportsmen.

The term "arthritis" means inflammation of a joint and usually involves a synovial joint. There are many causes, ranging from direct trauma to infection. Arthritis leads to a painful swelling of the joint which reduces the range of movement which may be undertaken. Long term, or chronic, arthritis leads to an alteration in the nature of the synovial fluid which loses its normal lubricant properties. In addition, there may be destruction of articular cartilage, with loss of the normal smooth surfaces, and these changes lead to a further reduction in joint function resulting from pain, friction and reduced range of movement.

The types of movement which may occur at synovial joints are:

(1) **Extension/Flexion**
    Extension increases the angle between bones ('straightens' the joint), whereas flexion reduces it ('bends' the joint).

(2) **Abduction/Adduction**
    Abduction carries the moving part (usually the limb) away from the midline of the body, whereas adduction brings the part towards the midline.

(3) **Circumduction**
    Movement of one end of a bone follows a circular pattern (Fig. 12-5).

Joint movement should be assessed in the conscious animal, since the muscles and soft tissues surrounding a joint normally constrain it. The range and type of movement that can be produced by manipulation of the joints in an anaesthetised animal is often far greater than that encountered in the conscious animal.

THE SKELETON

In considering the numerous components of the skeleton there is little to be gained from learning the name and position of all the bones in the body. It is far more useful to grasp an understanding of the position of those bones which are normally palpable in the living animal, and to be able to recognise the major bones on a radiograph. In this respect, it is useful to examine a dog or cat (or even yourself!), trying to locate and identify the structures described below. Similarly, reference to radiographs is very useful in helping to understand the position and articulation of bones.

THE AXIAL SKELETON

The axial skeleton comprises the skull, vertebral column and ribs.

The Skull
The skull is composed of a large number of bones, most of which join at fibrous joints, with little, if any movement between them. Most of the skull bones are flat bones. The major components are (Fig. 12-6):

162

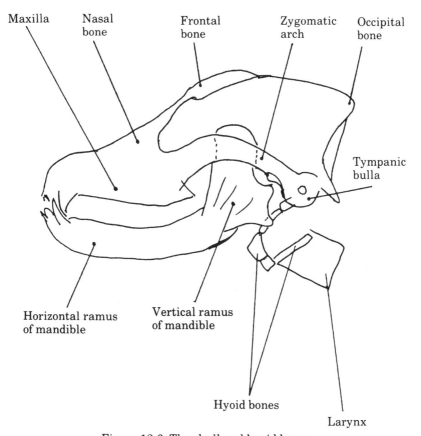

Maxilla   Nasal   Frontal   Zygomatic   Occipital
           bone   bone   arch   bone

Tympanic
bulla

Horizontal ramus   Vertical ramus
of mandible   of mandible

Hyoid bones

Larynx

Figure 12-6. The skull and hyoid bones.

The **mandible:** the lower jaw bone which articulates with part of the temporal bone at the tempero-mandibular joint. The mandible is divided into the horizontal ramus (which contains teeth) and the vertical ramus, which is the site of insertion of the main muscles of mastication.

The **maxilla, incisive** and **palatine** bones: together these make up the upper jaw, the hard palate and the floor of the nasal cavity.

The **nasal** bone: this forms the roof and lateral walls of the nasal cavity.

The **frontal** bone: this makes up part of the rostral wall of the cranium.

The **zygoma** bone: forms the zygomatic arch which runs from the maxilla, rostrally, to the temporal bone, caudally. It is easily palpated (the 'cheek-bone') as it forms part of the ventral and lateral walls of the orbit. The vertical ramus of the mandible lies medial to the zygomatic arch.

The **temporal** bone: although not palpable in the normal animal is recognised on radiographs by the characteristic bony enlargement, the tympanic bulla, which houses the middle ear.

163

The **occipital** bone: forms the caudal wall of the cranium; its dorsal part is the occipital protuberance and is normally palpable.

The **hyoid** bones: a collection of small bones, fashioned as a cradle, which run from the temporal bone to the larynx. They support the larynx, allowing it to move, primarily in the cranio-caudal direction, at the time of swallowing (Chapter 8).

The Vertebral Column

The vertebral column is composed of about 50 bones, or vertebrae, arranged in five sections. The vertebrae protect the delicate nervous tissue of the spinal cord which runs in the vertebral canal. They also provide sites for the attachment of muscles. As upright primates we tend to forget that the vertebral column is important in the locomotion of many quadrupeds, especially at speed – look at a greyhound carefully!

The features common to all vertebrae include a vertebral body with an overlying vertebral arch which surrounds the vertebral canal. Arising from the dorsal aspect of the vertebral arch is the spinous process. The transverse processes, by contrast, arise from the two sides of the vertebral body. These provide sites for the insertion of muscles (Fig. 12-7a).

At the articulation between vertebrae there are synovial joints between the articular processes on the vertebral arch. Lying between the vertebral bodies are intervertebral discs (Fig. 12-7b). These are roughly circular in cross-section, and consist of two regions:

(1) An outer fibrous layer, called the anulus fibrosus

(2) An inner gelatinous area, the nuclear pulposus.

The intervertebral disc serves as a shock absorber between the vertebrae, it also allows movement between the bones.

The tissue of the nucleus pulposus undergoes certain chemical and physical changes with age, with replacement of the gelatinous material by fibrous tissue plus cartilage. In addition, calcium may be laid down in the cartilage, so allowing the discs to be seen on radiographs.

Prolapse of an intervertebral disc (sometimes called a "slipped disc") involves the protrusion of disc material into the overlying vertebral canal. This places pressure on the spinal cord and often interferes with neurological function leading to paralysis. Prolapse of intervertebral discs is commoner in certain breeds of dog, e.g. Dachshunds and Spaniels, but it can occur in almost any breed.

The vertebral column is divided into five regions in which the vertebrae have certain distinguishing features.

Cervical Vertebrae (7 vertebrae)

The first two cervical vertebrae are modified to allow movements of the head. The first cervical vertebra is called the atlas (because in humans it carries the

164

A) Structure of a basic vertebra.

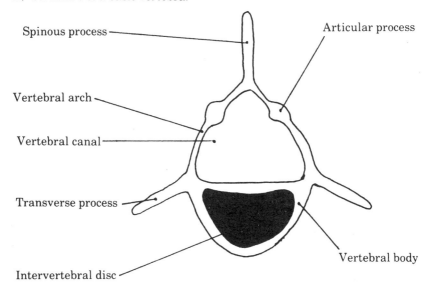

Spinous process

Articular process

Vertebral arch

Vertebral canal

Transverse process

Intervertebral disc

Vertebral body

B) Articulation between vertebrae.

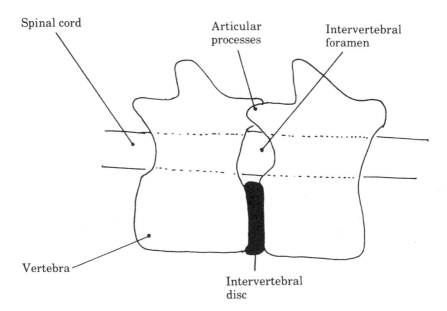

Spinal cord

Articular processes

Intervertebral foramen

Vertebra

Intervertebral disc

Figure 12-7.

skull as, in mythology, Atlas carried the world); it articulates with the base of the skull. Uniquely it has no vertebral body, but instead has two large lateral processes called wings; these are usually palpable in the conscious animal. The axis is the second cervical vertebra, it lies behind the atlas and has a short bony protrusion from the cranial end of the vertebral body called the odontoid peg. The vertebral arch of the axis is very large. The articulation between skull, atlas and axis allow the enormous range of head movements seen in normal animals.

The remaining five cervical vertebrae are all similar; they possess a strong vertebral arch, however, they have poorly developed spinous processes but stout transverse processes.

Thoracic Vertebrae (13 vertebrae)

The thoracic vertebrae have short vertebral bodies and prominent spinous processes, these may be felt when palpating the spine of a dog. Each thoracic vertebra articulates with a rib, by means of a synovial joint.

Lumbar Vertebrae (7 vertebrae)

Lumbar vertebrae have long vertebral bodies, compared with the thoracic vertebrae, but lack a distinct spinous process. There are large transverse processes which extend cranially and laterally, providing sites for the insertion of muscles, and also protecting the underlying kidneys. The extent to which they are palpable is the basis of 'condition scoring' of sheep.

Sacral Vertebrae (3 vertebrae)

The three vertebrae are fused in the adult to form the sacrum. This articulates with the ilium (part of the hip bone or pelvis) by means of a cartilaginous joint, the sacroiliac joint. This articulation allows mechanical forces to be efficiently transferred from the hindleg to the verterbal column.

Caudal Vertebrae (up to 20 vertebrae)

These are also called the coccygeal vertebrae, and the number present varies between breeds. These vertebrae support the tail.

The Ribs

The ribs support the lateral wall of the chest. Each rib is composed of a dorsal bony section which joins with a ventral cartilaginous section at the costo-chondral junction. The ribs are arranged in pairs, and each articulates with a thoracic vertebra dorsally. The cranial eight ribs (sometimes called the true ribs) articulate with the sternum ventrally, whereas the caudal five ribs do not articulate directly with the sternum, and are called the "floating ribs". The ribs provide extensive protection for the thorax (especially the heart and lungs) as well as providing a mechanical framework for its expansion during breathing (Chapter 3).

166

CRANIAL   CAUDAL

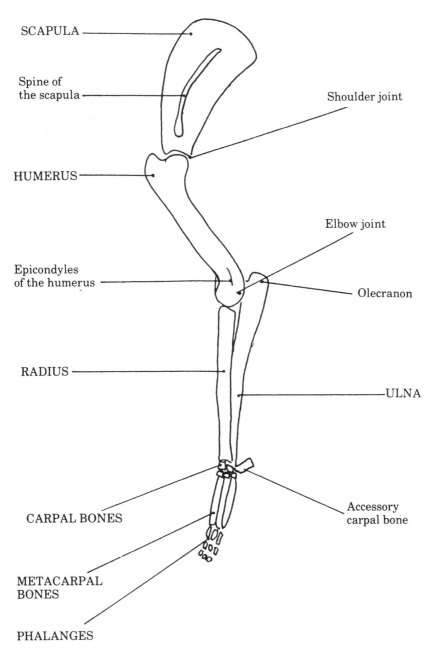

SCAPULA

Spine of
the scapula   Shoulder joint

HUMERUS

                                           Elbow joint

Epicondyles
of the humerus   Olecranon

RADIUS   ULNA

CARPAL BONES   Accessory
                                           carpal bone

METACARPAL
BONES

PHALANGES

Figure 12-8. The bones of the forelimb.

167

THE APPENDICULAR SKELETON

This is the skeleton of the limbs.

The Forelimb (Fig. 12-8)

There is no bony connection between the forelimb and the trunk in domestic animals, unlike the situation in man where the clavicle (collar bone) forms a rigid strut between the shoulder joint and the sternum. This probably reflects the difference between primates – which predominantly move using their hindlegs or by swinging from their arms – and quadrupeds which continuously need a shock-absorbing system at the front end, especially if they gallop or jump. The spine of the scapula is often palpable on its lateral surface and extends down almost to the shoulder joint. This is a hinge joint between the scapula and humerus and much support is provided by the adjacent muscles.

The clavicle is poorly developed in domestic animals though it is normally present in the cat, and sometimes present in the dog. It is a small bone which lies in the muscles just cranial to the shoulder joint. It may be seen on radiographs of the shoulder region.

The distal part of the humerus is usually palpable; you can feel the two epicondyles which lie just above the articular regions, called the condyles. The distal humerus articulates with both the radius and ulna at the elbow joint, which permits flexion and extension. The ulna lies caudal to the radius at the elbow, and is easily palpated at the olecranon (or point of the elbow). Moving distally along the forearm, the relationship of the radius to the ulna alters, so that the radius comes to lie medial to the ulna, and both bones are normally palpable in the distal forearm. The ulna of the cat is a more substantial bone compared with that of the dog.

The carpus (wrist) is made up of two rows of short bones. It is a complex joint, and allows articulation between the distal forearm and the metacarpus. Individual bones of the carpus are rarely palpable, except for the accessory carpal bone which lies on the caudal and lateral surface of the carpus.

Articulating with the distal row of carpal bones are the five metacarpal bones. The first metacarpal bone lies medially, and is very small in the dog and cat. It forms part of the dew claw (Chapter 2). The four main metacarpal bones are normally palpable from the dorsal surface of the limb. These metacarpal bones articulate with the proximal phalanx of a digit. Each digit has three phalanges, the distal phalanx being partly covered by the claw (Chapter 2). The bones of the digits are most easily palpated from the dorsal surface, since their palmar surface is covered, in part, by the foot pads (Chapter 2).

The Hindlimb (Figs. 12-9; 12-10)

Unlike the forelimb, there is a rigid connection between the hindlimb and the vertebral column, by means of the sacroiliac joint.

The hip bone is made up of three bones, the ilium, ischium and pubis, fused together. The wing of the ilium is normally palpable, lateral to the vertebral

CRANIAL

ILIUM

PUBIS

Acetabulum

Obturator
foramen

Pelvic
symphysis

Ischial
tuberosity

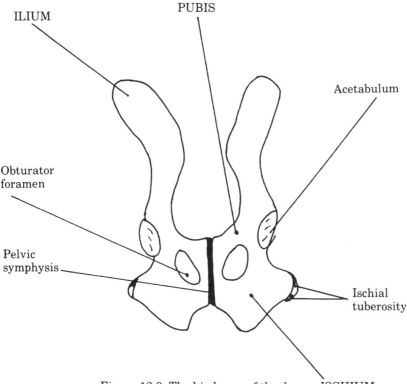

Figure 12-9. The hip bones of the dog.   ISCHIUM
(Ventral view)

column. The ischium lies more caudally, and a prominence, the ischial
tuberosity, is normally palpable lateral and ventral to the anus. The third
component of the hip bone is the pubis, which is positioned more ventrally and
can be palpated in the region of the groin. The two hip bones meet at the pubic
symphysis, a cartilaginous joint, and lying lateral to this is a large hole, the
obturator foramen. This is clearly visible on radiographs made for the
assessment of hip dysplasia. As a whole, the pelvis provides a protective
enclosure for various organs including the bladder and, until advanced
pregnancy, part of the uterus (this varies with species).

The ilium, ischium and pubis all meet at the acetabulum. This is a deep cavity
which articulates with the head of the femur to form the hip joint. A small
ligament runs in the joint from the centre of the acetabulum to the head of the
femur. Extension and flexion, and abduction and adduction are all possible at
the hip joint, because of its 'ball and socket' shape.

The great trochanter, a bony prominence on the lateral aspect of the proximal
femur, is often palpable in the conscious animal; it serves as the site for the
insertion of the gluteal muscles.

169

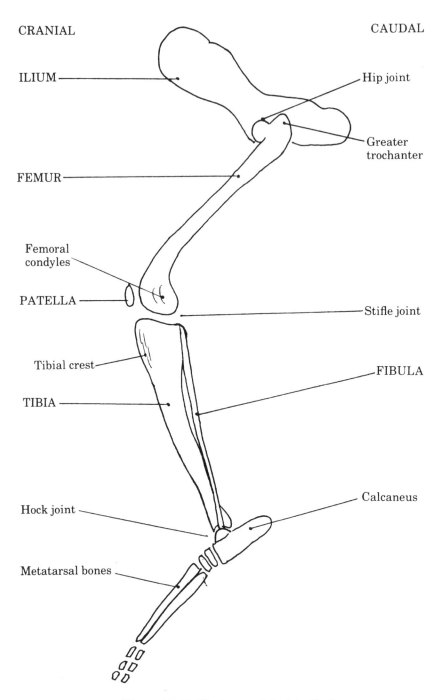

CRANIAL

CAUDAL

ILIUM

Hip joint

Greater trochanter

FEMUR

Femoral condyles

PATELLA

Stifle joint

Tibial crest

FIBULA

TIBIA

Calcaneus

Hock joint

Metatarsal bones

Figure 12-10. The bones of the hindlimb.

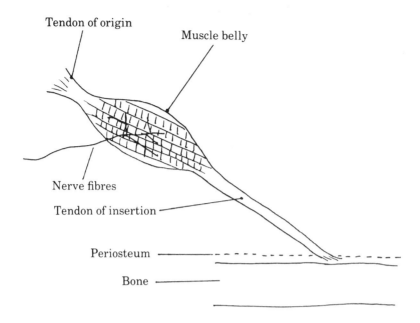

Tendon of origin

Muscle belly

Nerve fibres

Tendon of insertion

Periosteum

Bone

Figure 12-11. Structure of a muscle.

At the distal femur, the lateral and medial condyles are normally palpable. Lying cranial to them is the patella (kneecap) which lies in a small groove, the trochlea. A radiograph of the stifle reveals two, or often three, small sesamoid bones lying in the muscles caudal to the stifle joint. Movement at the stifle joint normally involves extension and flexion.

The femur articulates with the tibia and fibula at the stifle joint. The fibula is a thin, almost stick-like bone, which lies lateral to the much larger tibia. Proximally, the tibia is expanded to form the tibial crest which is easily palpated on the cranial surface of the leg. Distally, the tibia and fibula articulate with the bones of the hock.

The hock joint, like the carpus, is composed of numerous short bones, arranged in three rows. Movement is normally restricted to extension and flexion between the distal tibia and the proximal row of tarsal bones. The calcaneus extends caudally from the hock joint to form the point of the hock which is the site of insertion of the Achilles tendon, and is easily palpable.

The arrangement of the metatarsal bones and phalanges is very similar to the arrangement of the metacarpal bones described for the forelimb. However, it is uncommon for the first digit to be present in the hindfoot.

THE MUSCULAR SYSTEM

The bulk of the body's muscle mass is skeletal muscle, also called striated or voluntary muscle; smooth muscle and cardiac muscle are described below.

171

Skeletal muscles play an important role in locomotion as well as providing support and protection for the limbs and for the body cavities, e.g. the abdominal wall described in Chapter 8. In Chapter 3 the importance of skeletal muscles in breathing was emphasised, and must always be considered when using muscle relaxant drugs. Finally, shivering, or the involuntary contraction of skeletal muscle, results in production of heat.

A muscle is made up of a belly plus its tendons of insertion and origin (Fig. 12-11). The belly contains many muscle cells, or fibres, held together by connective tissue. In addition, both nerves and blood vessels pass into or through the muscle belly.

Tendons attach muscle to bone. They are made of strands of collagen and have a glistening white appearance. They are very strong structures, but are also slightly elastic and act as shock absorbers in the musculoskeletal system. Where tendons pass over bony prominences there is a potential for them to be damaged by friction. This is prevented by the development of a fluid-filled cavity, called a bursa, which acts as a cushion between the tendon and the underlying bone. In some areas, the bursa is actually wrapped around the tendon, forming a tendon sheath.

In some muscles there is no discrete tendon of insertion but instead a broad sheet of fibrous tissue called an aponeurosis; examples are found in the muscles of the abdominal and thoracic walls.

Muscles are not able to function correctly without:

1. Efferent nerve supply

2. Mechanoreceptors; located in muscle fibres and tendons, and which detect alterations in the load applied to the muscle.

3. Blood, supplied by blood vessels, which themselves contain smooth muscle in their wall.

Maintenance of muscle mass is dependent upon its continuous function. If the efferent nerve to a muscle is damaged, for example in radial paralysis (Chapter 10) there will be atrophy, or wasting, of the muscles served by that nerve. Similarly, if a leg is placed in a plaster cast, it will not be used properly, and within a few weeks the cast will loosen due to atrophy of muscle. Conversely, the response to a sustained workload is hypertrophy, an increased muscle mass.

There is little to be gained from attempting to learn the names and position of all the muscles of the body; it is far more useful to concentrate on understanding those which are of greatest clinical importance.

MUSCLES OF THE HEAD

The masseter and temporal muscles lie caudal to the orbit and medial to the zygomatic arch. They pass from the skull to the mandible and act to close the jaw. Occasionally they become inflamed (myositis) and this leads to difficulty in opening the jaw. The tongue is a complex mass of muscle used for obtaining and swallowing food; it has been discussed in more detail in Chapter 8.

172

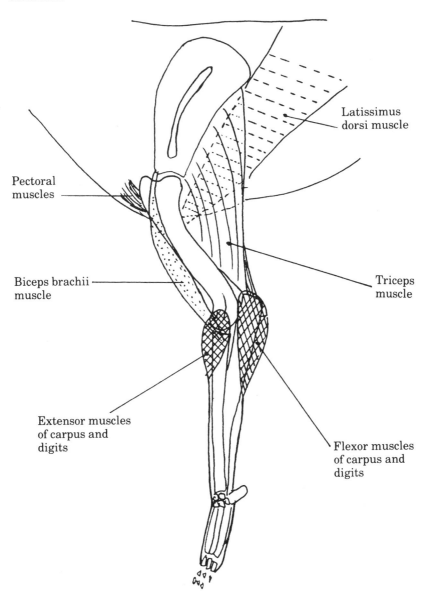

Latissimus dorsi muscle

Pectoral muscles

Biceps brachii muscle

Triceps muscle

Extensor muscles of carpus and digits

Flexor muscles of carpus and digits

Figure 12-12. Muscles of the forelimb.

Within the orbit are several small muscles attaching to the outside of the eye (extraocular muscles); they are responsible for producing movements of the eye. Contraction of the superficial muscles of the head alters facial expression and ear position (Chapter 11).

MUSCLES OF THE TRUNK

Muscles lie dorsal and ventral to the vertebral column, providing support and protection for it. These muscles also produce movement in the spine. Movement and flexibility of the spine is very important for efficient locomotion in animals. The diaphragm, intercostal muscles and the muscles of the abdominal wall have all been described in Chapters 3 and 8.

MUSCLES OF THE LIMBS

Two major categories of limb muscles are recognised. Extrinsic muscles originate at the trunk, and insert on the limb bones, whereas intrinsic muscles both originate and insert in the limb. Contraction of extrinsic muscles causes movement of the limb with respect to the trunk, whereas contraction of intrinsic muscles leads to movement of bones within the limb.

The Forelimb (Fig. 12-2)

The latissimus dorsi is a large, fan-shaped extrinsic muscle which runs from the thoracic vertebrae, over the wall of the chest, to insert on the humerus. Not only is this muscle important for locomotion, it also provides protection for the underlying thoracic cavity.

The pectoral muscles run from the medial surface of the humerus to the sternum. They play a role in locomotion and also hold the forelimb close to the trunk, preventing excessive abduction.

The triceps muscle lies caudal to the humerus, running from the scapula to insert on the olecranon. It extends the elbow joint. The radial nerve (Chapter 10) runs through the triceps muscle. The biceps brachii muscle lies on the cranial surface of the humerus, passing from the scapula and inserting onto the proximal ulna. It flexes the elbow joint.

Overlying the proximal radius and ulna are several groups of muscles whose site of action is the carpus and digits. These muscles have relatively long tendons of insertion. Those lying cranially and laterally act as extensors of the carpus and digits, those positioned more caudally and medially are the flexors of the carpus and digit.

The Hindlimb (Fig. 12-13)

The quadriceps femoris muscle has origins at both the ilium and proximal femur, and runs on the cranial surface of the femur. It inserts onto the tibial crest, by means of the patellar tendon, which contains the patella (a sesamoid bone). This muscle is the main extensor of the stifle. The gluteals are a group of muscles which runs from the hip bone to the greater trochanter. They extend the hip joint.

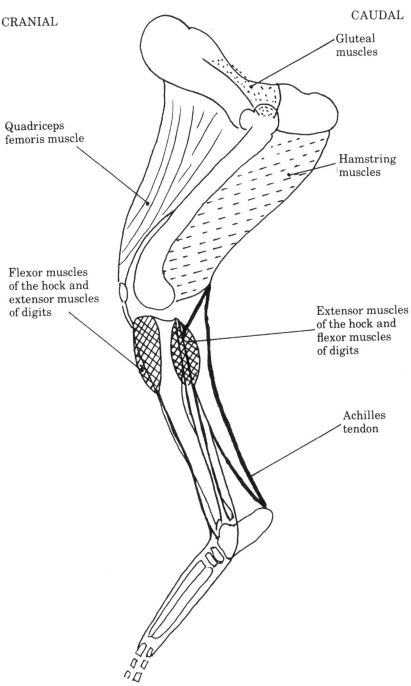

CRANIAL

CAUDAL

Gluteal muscles

Quadriceps femoris muscle

Hamstring muscles

Flexor muscles of the hock and extensor muscles of digits

Extensor muscles of the hock and flexor muscles of digits

Achilles tendon

Figure 12-13. Muscles of the hindlimb.

175

A group of three large muscles, the 'hamstrings' (biceps femoris, semimembranosus and semitendinosus), lies on the caudal aspect of the femur, originating at the ischial arch and inserting on the distal femur, proximal tibia and the calcaneus. They are responsible for extending the hip, and are important in locomotion since the thrust generated by their contraction will push the body forward. The sciatic nerve (Chapter 10) runs through the hamstring muscles.

Muscle groups lying on the cranial surface of the proximal tibia flex the hock joint and extend the digits. Again, these muscles have long tendons which pass down the limb to the point of insertion. Lying on the caudal aspect of the proximal tibia are muscles which act as extensors of the hock and flexors of the digits. The tendons of all the hock extensor muscles insert on the calcaneus as the Achilles tendon; this is easily palpable beneath the skin. Disruption of the Achilles tendon leads to loss of support for the hock which collapses as soon as weight is borne by the affected leg.

So far we have taken it for granted that muscles contract as and when necessary; now we need to wonder how – and how the precision of movement is achieved.

HOW MUSCLE MOVES

We understand best how skeletal muscle works. It is also called striated (striped) muscle because of its appearance under the microscope where we can see that each tiny fibre is made up of even smaller fibrils and that every fibril has alternating dark and light bands. These bands give the 'striped' appearance under the microscope, like an elongated sleeve of a rugby shirt.

A mixture of chemistry and electron-microscopy revealed that this appearance reflected the underlying arrangement of two types of microfilaments and that this, in turn, provided the basis of muscular contraction and, therefore, of movement.

The thin filaments (made of actin) lie between the thick filaments in a three-dimensional lattice – as if we had a regular pattern of thin and thick trees in a forest. But this is most easily visualised as a two-dimensional diagram (Fig. 12-14). In this, however, we have drawn an analogy with boat-race boats (myosin) lying between floating telegraph poles (actin) in order to illustrate how movement occurs.

Myosin has side-arms (you can see them with an electron-microscope) which spontaneously tend to attach to actin. These are the oars of the boats and we must imagine that the tips of the oars can attach to the poles. The diagram shows (left) two boat-race boats set to row in opposite directions (the top one towards the top of the page, the bottom one towards the bottom). Both begin with their oars attached to the adjacent poles and both boats are anchored so that when the crews row the oars move, but not the boats. What happens? Ready, go! The boats do not move (right) but the oars (side arms) do and so do the poles attached to them; the poles at the top and bottom (actin) slide towards one another and the distance between the ends of each pair of poles (X) is shortened; there has been contraction. If, at the end of the stroke, the

176

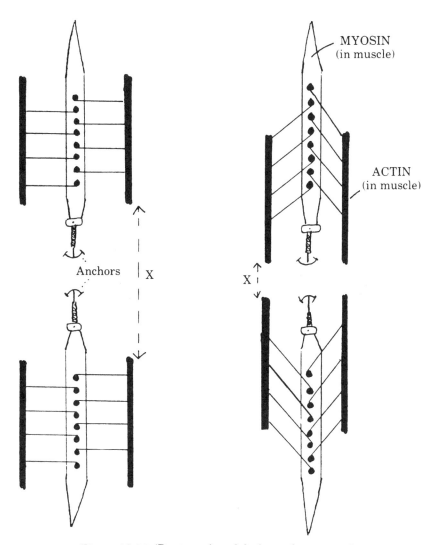

Figure 12-14. 'Boat-race' model of muscle contraction.

oars detach from the poles and the crews move into position for the next stroke, allowing the oars to attach again to the poles, the next stroke will move the poles even closer together, causing even greater 'contraction'.

Because the thick filaments can move the thin filaments in this way, making them slide between, the fibrils as a whole contract and so does the muscle as a whole. It is the detachment of the side-arms from the actin (oars from poles) that actually needs energy (ATP); the tendency to attach is spontaneous. This is seen when the muscle runs out of ATP completely – at death; rigor mortis results from this spontaneous attachment (and only passes off as the muscle's

177

structure starts to break down completely). A struggle before death consumes ATP and rigor occurs faster. A muscle could not work long on its ATP stores; these have to be replenished from creatine phosphate (another energy store) and by utilising stored glycogen to generate ATP, both anaerobically and aerobically (Chapter 3). Much of the respiratory effort *after* exertion is to replenish depleted energy stores ('oxygen debt').

All we need to ask now is what gives the signal to start the movement? The nerve impulses reach a special sort of synapse with the muscle (an end plate) and the transmitter chemical depolarises the membranes of the muscle fibrils (which have a resting voltage, just like nerves). This causes a release of calcium within the fibrils and this, in its turn, causes the movement of a protein which normally lies between the side arms and actin to prevent attachment: in effect, the muscle is switched on by calcium (hence some of the problems in milk fever when blood calcium levels are inadequate). When movement stops the calcium is pumped back into storage within the muscle until it is needed to trigger the next 'twitch'.

PRECISION OF MOVEMENT

The end branches of a nerve fibre may trigger very few end plates or very many and therefore cause very few fibrils or very many fibrils to contract simultaneously; such a cluster of fibrils, contracting together, is called a motor unit. A muscle with relatively few motor units made up of large number of fibrils would tend to give relatively powerful contractions but with little gradation of strength. With more motor units, each less powerful (fewer fibrils) we could gain a gradation of strength of contraction, according to how many motor units were stimulated at once. Strength of contraction rests on numbers of fibrils called into play, not on changes in how strongly each contracts.

If we turn to whole muscle, the limb muscles seldom act singly. The nervous system produces co-ordinated contraction of groups of muscles, often opposing groups. Thus when the flexors bend a joint there is controlled slight opposition from the extensors allowing finer overall control of the movement – rather like using clutch and brake in parking a car in an awkward space.

How does the animal 'know' (subconsciously) how much the muscle is contracting or how fast? There are very special stretch receptors (muscle spindles) within the muscle. The system is very sophisticated because they too are innervated and they too have special muscle fibres so that the nervous system can adjust how tense or relaxed, and therefore how sensitive they are. This is part of the basis of the resting 'tone' of a muscle – limb muscles are seldom fully relaxed unless an animal is deeply asleep or anaesthetised. Naturally when an animal stands, the muscle tone is considerable even though the muscle stays stationary. In fact muscles undergo two types of contraction: isotonic – where they actually cause movement, or isometric – where they simply generate tension – as in pressing down on a table. Normal limb movements in walking involve alternating phases of both.

There are also stretch receptors in tendons and stretch receptors in joint capsules. There is thus a wealth of information reaching the CNS which

178

allows it to interpret and control, subconsciously, the exact position of the various limbs and the speed and direction of any movements. So even with our eyes shut, it is easy to put the tip of a finger on the end of our nose! This co-ordination is vital, not just for smooth and effective movement but because the limb muscles are so powerful that wrongly co-ordinated movements (e.g. during bad recovery from anaesthesia, especially in horses) can tear tendons away from bones or even cause fractures. Inco-ordinate contractions of limb muscles produce 'convulsions' (seizures, fits) which may be 'clonic' (paddling movements) or 'tonic' (spasms).

Obviously skeletal muscle only contracts when triggered by nerves; it has no spontaneous rhythm of contraction. This is in contrast with the other two types of muscle; smooth and cardiac.

SMOOTH MUSCLE: CARDIAC MUSCLE

Smooth muscle, found in the blood vessels and viscera (gut, bladder, glands, uterus, etc), does not look striped under the microscope whereas cardiac muscle does. Smooth muscle often has a spontaneous rhythm of contraction, though this rhythm can be controlled by nerves. Cardiac muscle always has a spontaneous rhythm of contraction – even cardiac muscle cells in the embryo, before the heart is properly formed. The spontaneous rhythm of the ventricles is very slow so they are normally paced from the AV node (Chapter 6) but if this fails (as in heart block) they do not simply stop. The region of the heart with the fastest spontaneous rhythm obviously sets the overall pace of the heart: normally this is towards the top of the right atrium where the sinoatrial node acts as the natural pacemaker. Its frequency is altered by neural activity (Chapter 6). So the sinoatrial node dictates the contraction frequency of the normal heart – it is said to be 'in sinus rhthym'. Damaged heart muscle can act as an abnormal pacemaker, generating extra or 'ectopic' beats (extrasystoles).

179

CHAPTER 13:
THE REPRODUCTIVE SYSTEM

All living species, be they bacteria, tapeworms or dogs and cats must reproduce if they are to survive. Reproduction in mammals is a complex process, and in these animals certain areas of the body are specialised for reproduction; these areas make up the genital system.

Certain parts of the genital system are shared with the urinary system and a revision of Chapter 7 may be useful at this point.

Essentially reproductive physiology can be viewed in three phases.

(a) **The events leading to fertilisation**
These comprise the oestrous cycle of the female (which co-ordinates the availability of ova for fertilisation with sexual receptiveness), the formation of sperm in the male, together with mating and fertilisation.

(b) **Pregnancy**
The events from fertilisation of an ovum by a sperm through to the emergence of a foetus at birth (parturition).

(c) **Lactation**
This is a period when not only do the offspring receive nutritional support from their mother, in the form of milk, they are also protected, kept warm and, increasingly as the period progresses, they learn a lot from her (including, in the wild, much of their hunting/feeding behaviour).

Since the male is only involved in fertilisation it is convenient to begin there, and continue with the female.

THE MALE

THE TESTIS

The gonad is that part of the genital system responsible for producing the gametes, or sex cells. The male gonad is the testis and it produces the male sex cell, the sperm. Like the ovum, the sperm has half the normal adult number of

CRANIAL   CAUDAL

Testicular   Bladder   Prostate   Urethra   Rectum
blood vessels   gland

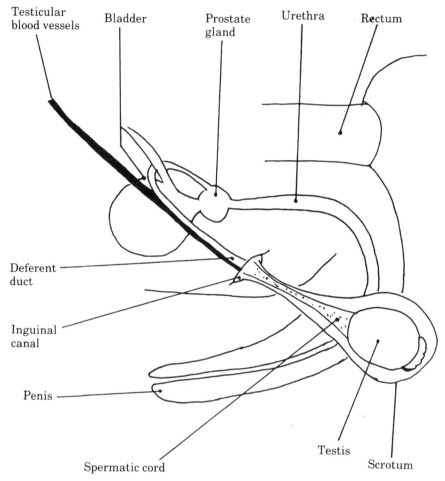

Deferent
duct

Inguinal
canal

Penis

                                              Testis
         Spermatic cord   Scrotum

Figure 13-1. Longitudinal section of the pelvis of the dog to demonstrate the
         genital tract.

chromosomes (i.e. it is a 'haploid') so that at fertilisation, when the nuclei of
the two gametes fuse, the normal adult number (diploid) is restored and each
pair of chromosomes contains one originating from each gamete. The special
form of cell division which halves the number of chromosomes in producing
the gametes is 'meiosis' ('reduction division') in contrast to normal cell
division (mitosis) in which the number of chromosomes stays constant.

The testes are paired, oval-shaped structures which, in the adult, lie in the
scrotum, a small sac of almost hairless skin, lying ventral to the bony pelvis
(Fig. 13-1). The testes are normally palpable through the scrotal skin and are
quite mobile within the scrotum. Each testis is composed of a large number of

182

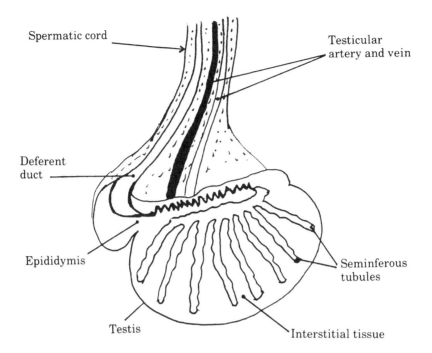

Spermatic cord

Testicular artery and vein

Deferent duct

Epididymis

Seminiferous tubules

Testis

Interstitial tissue

Figure 13-2. The structure of the testis.

blind-ending ducts, the seminiferous tubules (Fig. 13-2). Cells lining the tubules produce sperm. Sperm production, or spermatogenesis, is a continuous process, commencing at the time of puberty and it lacks the markedly cyclical pattern seen with ovulation in the female. Between the seminiferous tubules lies the interstitial tissue which contains fibrous tissue and interstitial cells; the latter produce testosterone (Chapter 8). The testis is covered by a layer of peritoneum which is continuous with the parietal peritoneum of the abdomen (Chapter 6). This peritoneal layer is often called the vaginal tunic of the testis.

Sperm are small cells which have a head, body and tail (Fig. 13-3). The tail is responsible for the inherent motility of these cells which is easily seen if a sample of semen is examined under the microscope.

In the embryo the testes develop within the abdomen, close to the kidneys. During the later stages of embryonic development they migrate across the abdominal cavity, taking their blood supply with them, and pass out through the inguinal canal. This is one of the "normal" openings of the abdominal wall (Chapter 8) and lies in the caudolateral part of the wall, near to the groin.

Sperm formation (spermatogenesis) begins at puberty and is influenced by many factors including the ambient temperature; increasing the temperature inhibits sperm production. The temperature in the scrotum is less than core body temperature and this arrangement allows favourable

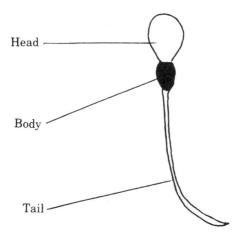

Head

Body

Tail

Figure 13-3. The structure of a sperm.

conditions for spermatogenesis. In some animals, referred to as cryptorchids, one, or sometimes both, testes fail to descend correctly into the scrotum and are retained either in the abdominal cavity or in the inguinal canal. The retained testis is of little use to the animal since it does not produce sperm correctly. Perhaps more worrying is the knowledge that the retained testis is quite likely to become neoplastic later in life.

THE EPIDIDYMIS

The epididymis is a convoluted structure positioned on the dorsal and caudal borders of the testis (Fig. 13-2). It stores sperm until they pass up the deferent duct. The tail of the epididymis is normally palpable through the scrotal skin as a distinct raised region lying on the caudal border of the testis.

THE DEFERENT DUCT

This is a fibromuscular tube which passes from the epididymis up through the inguinal canal into the abdomen where it runs through the prostate gland to enter the urethra (Fig. 13-1).

As sperm pass from the seminiferous tubules into the epididymis and along the deferent duct they mature, becoming capable of fertilising the female gametes, or ova. The time taken for maturation of sperm in the dog is up to 8 weeks.

THE SPERMATIC CORD

The spermatic cord runs from the testis to the inguinal canal. It is a composite structure, with an outer covering of peritoneum, beneath which lies the deferent duct, the testicular artery and vein, lymphatic vessels and a small strip of muscle called the cremaster muscle. The testicular artery and vein carry blood to and from the testis. The testicular artery arises from the aorta, just caudal to the kidneys, and the testicular vein joins the caudal vena cava in the same area.

THE PROSTATE GLAND

The prostate is an accessory sexual gland. It surrounds the proximal urethra, lying just caudal to the bladder (Fig. 13-1). The development and function of the prostate gland is influenced by testosterone. At puberty, the period of attainment of sexual maturity, there is an increase in size of the gland. Secretions produced by the prostate pass into the urethra and neutralise any residual acidity due to urine remaining there. The secretions are also a source of nutrients for sperm.

The prostate gland can usually be palpated by introducing a gloved finger into the rectum. The prostate lies ventral to the rectum. Enlargement of the prostate is not uncommon in middle-aged dogs, and it may compress the overlying rectum, causing constipation, or may place pressure on the urethra, leading to difficulty in urinating (dysuria).

THE PENIS

The penis is composed of specialised erectile vascular tissue, the size and stiffness of which may be increased by alterations in local blood flow. Penile wounds, be they either surgical, e.g. at the time of urethrotomy, or traumatic will bleed profusely since there is damage to the erectile tissue. At its base, the penis is attached by muscles and ligaments to the ischium, part of the bony pelvis. The penis of the dog and cat (but not the penis of the horse, bull or man) contains a small supporting bone, the os penis. The urethra, which is the common outflow tract for both the genital and urinary systems, lies in the penis ventral to the os penis (Fig. 7-4).

In the dog the penis lies ventral to the pelvis, and extends cranially, whereas in the cat it is directed caudally, opening ventral to the anus (Fig. 7-5). The distal part of the penis is called the glans penis; this is relatively mobile compared with the more proximal base of the penis. In the tomcat the glans penis has numerous sharp barbs on its surface which are thought to stimulate the queen's vagina at the time of mating. At the time of sexual arousement, and at copulation, or mating, blood supply to the erectile tissue of the penis increases, causing it to enlarge and stiffen. The glans penis protrudes from the overlying prepuce through the preputial orifice. The prepuce is a tubular fold of skin which overlies and protects the penis. The preputial orifice lies at its distal end (Fig. 7-4).

THE FEMALE

THE OVARY

The female gonads are the ovaries, paired structures which lie in the abdomen, just caudal to the kidneys (Fig. 13-5). They produce the female gametes, or ova (singular: ovum) and they also produce hormones (Chapter 9). Each ovary contains many fluid-filled follicles, and in each follicle there is a

185

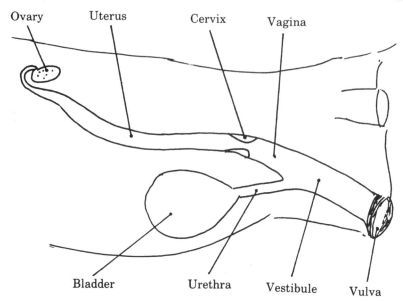

CRANIAL   CAUDAL

Ovary   Uterus   Cervix   Vagina

Bladder   Urethra   Vestibule   Vulva

Figure 13-4. Longitudinal section of the caudal abdomen and pelvis to demonstrate the genital tract of the bitch.

developing ovum. The ova are formed before birth but they only mature, a few at a time, during oestrous cycles. From the time of puberty there is regular development and enlargement of follicles, with the subsequent release of a mature ovum from the surface of the ovary, a process called ovulation. In dogs and cats there is usually simultaneous release of a number of ova at ovulation, whereas in women only one ovum is normally released. Following ovulation there is formation of a corpus luteum at the site of the ruptured follicle, and this is responsible for production of progesterone (Chapter 9).

Most animals, including the bitch, are "spontaneous ovulators". Ovulation occurs independent of mating (copulation). The result is that many ova will be wasted since they will not be fertilised. By contrast, "induced ovulators" need vaginal stimulation at the time of copulation to cause the release of ova. The co-ordination of ovulation involves both nervous and hormonal pathways. Cats and rabbits are induced ovulators and their release of ova is thus synchronised to the presence of sperm in the genital tract, providing optimal conditions for successful fertilisation.

The ovaries are supported within the abdominal cavity by special folds of peritoneum, called the mesovarium. This is wrapped around the ovary to form a small sac called the ovarian bursa. It is common for fat to be deposited in the mesovarium, so the ovary is not clearly seen when examining the genital tract during surgery, especially in the bitch.

186

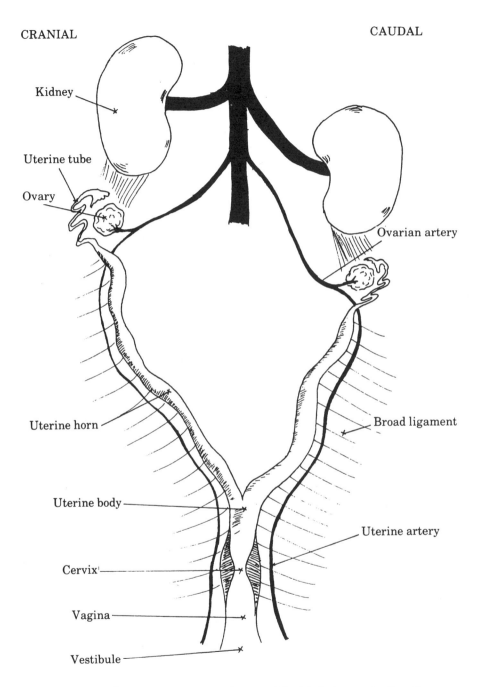

CRANIAL

CAUDAL

Kidney

Uterine tube

Ovary

Ovarian artery

Uterine horn

Broad ligament

Uterine body

Uterine artery

Cervix

Vagina

Vestibule

Figure 13-5. Dorsal view of the genital tract of the bitch demonstrating the blood supply to the uterus.

187

THE UTERINE TUBE

Ova released from the surface of the ovary pass into the open end of a small, convoluted tube, the uterine tube (Fig. 13-5). (This is sometimes called the oviduct, or fallopian tube.) It runs caudally to join the uterine horn. In the bitch the uterine tube is often obscured by overlying fat.

Fertilisation, penetration of an ovum by a sperm, occurs in the uterine tube. However, because the journey from ovary to oviduct crosses a minute gap which is simply part of the peritoneal cavity, it can occasionally happen that a fertilised ovum starts its development in the abdominal cavity instead of the uterus; such a pregnancy is doomed.

THE UTERUS

The uterus is a Y-shaped tubular structure situated in the abdomen. It is composed of two horns and a body (Figs. 13-4; 13-5). The uterus has a glandular lining and its walls contain smooth muscle, which is called the myometrium. Embryos develop in the uterus prior to being expelled from the animal at parturition. Secretions produced by the uterine glands serve in the early nutrition of the embryo, before the development of the placenta. Development and activity of the glands is under hormonal control. The size of the uterus is very variable. It enlarges during pregnancy so as to accommodate the growing embryos. Contraction of the myometrium is responsible for the forceful expulsion of the mature foetus at parturition.

The uterus is supported in the abdomen by a fold of peritoneum called the broad ligament, or mesometrium, which contains a variable amount of fat. Blood vessels supplying the uterus run in the broad ligament. The uterus has a dual blood supply (Fig. 13-5). The ovarian artery is a paired vessel which arises from the aorta just caudal to the kidneys, and supplies the ovary and the horn of the uterus. It anastomoses with the uterine artery which supplies the more caudal sections of the uterus. The blood supply to the uterus increases as the uterus enlarges. In many species (but not cats, dogs or humans) the uterus is also an endocrine gland, producing certain prostaglandins which contribute to the regulation of the oestrous cycle by limiting the life of the corpora lutea.

THE CERVIX

The body of the uterus leads into the cervix caudally (Fig. 13-4). This is a thick-walled tubular structure which acts as a sphincter, controlling the opening into the uterus. It is normally closed, so sealing and protecting the uterus. However, at certain times it relaxes and opens. These include:

1. At oestrus, to allow the entry of sperm

2. At parturition, to allow the expulsion of foetuses.

Since the uterus, via the oviduct, is a potential access to the peritoneal cavity (see above) the cervix is not only vital in protecting the uterus (and the foetus) from pathogens but also the peritoneum. The uterine wall also becomes rich in white cells (defence cells) just after oestrus, as seen from vaginal smears.

188

THE VAGINA AND VESTIBULE

The vagina is a highly distensible canal running caudally from the cervix to the vestibule. At the time of copulation, the glans penis is introduced into the vagina and sperm are deposited here. The vestibule is a short passage which is shared by the genital and urinary systems. It is continuous with the vagina cranially, and runs caudoventrally to open at the vulva. The urethra opens onto the ventral floor of the vestibule (Fig. 13-4) near to the junction of vagina and vestibule. The lips, or labiae, of the vulva contain skeletal muscle and help to keep the vulva sealed.

The cell types present in the vaginal epithelium change during the oestrous cycle, being influenced by the circulating levels of oestrogen and progesterone. Swabs of vaginal epithelium can be examined with a microscope to determine the most appropriate time to mate the animal.

THE OESTROUS CYCLE

Once they are sexually mature, i.e. after puberty, the bitch or queen regularly shows a definite breeding season. During this season there are limited periods of sexual receptivity (or oestrus) when the female will accept the male. This is, of course, quite different from the situation in humans. On the other hand in most species (including dog and man) males remain sexually active throughout the year (though stags, for example, have a 'rutting' season). The rhythm of the cycle is controlled by the hypothalamus, acting on the anterior pituitary gland and regulating the release of its hormones (Chapter 9). It is, however, a dialogue since the hormones from the ovary both respond to the anterior pituitary hormones and help to regulate them, by 'feedback'. As the follicles mature they produce oestrogens which not only induce oestrous behaviour but also the surge of LH needed for ovulation. The high levels of oestrogen suppress further release of FSH (Chapter 9) so no more follicles ripen until the next cycle (another example of negative feedback: Fig. 13-6). Remember, all normal females have cycles; in seasonal breeders they are restricted to particular times of year, unlike non-seasonal breeders (e.g. cows).

THE BITCH

The bitch has only one period of oestrus during each breeding season and generally two seasons per year. The periods of the oestrous cycle are:

1. **Pro-oestrus:** The vulva enlarges and swells. The bitch's behaviour changes; she tends to roam and is more attractive to dogs; so is her urine (pheromones, Chapter 11). There is a vaginal discharge which contains blood. (This must not be confused with menstruation in women, where blood comes from the uterus at the end of the luteal phase.) In the ovaries there is rapid growth of many follicles, with maturation of the ova in them.

   Pro-oestrus lasts from 5 to 15 days, and the signs observed will vary between animals.

189

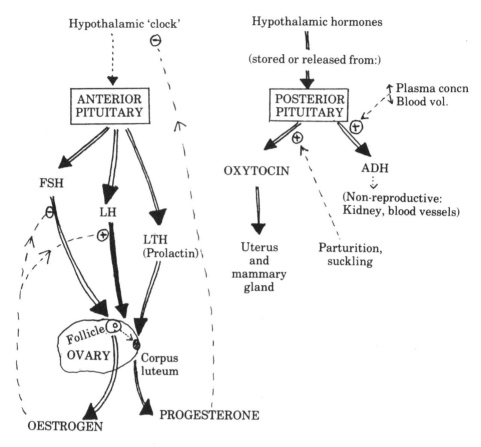

Figure 13-6. Pituitary and reproductive hormones.

2. **Oestrus:** This is the period of sexual receptivity when a bitch will stand for a dog. The vaginal discharge during this period is normally clear. Ovulation occurs during oestrus. 'Silent heat' refers to ovulation in the absence of obvious signs of oestrus.

Oestrus terminates when the bitch will no longer stand for the dog; it is of variable length, anywhere between 5 and 15 days. It is followed either by dioestrus or pregnancy.

3a. **Dioestrus:** (luteal phase). The period of progesterone domination of the genital tract, progresterone being produced by the corpora lutea in the ovaries (and later from the placenta if pregnancy occurs). The uterus undergoes development in preparation for implantation of the zygotes (fused gametes). Indeed many features resembling pregnancy may occur even without fertilisation (see 'false pregnancy', below).

Dioestrus lasts up to 70 days and ends when the corpora lutea regress and progesterone levels fall. It is followed by anoestrus.

190

3b. **Pseudopregnancy,** or false pregnancy, is not uncommon in the bitch following oestrus. During dioestrus there is development of corpora lutea in the ovary, with subsequent production of progesterone. The result, from an endocrinological viewpoint, is quite similar to that seen during pregnancy, indeed there can be real problems in distinguishing the two, even by hormone assay. Progesterone has been described as the "hormone of pregnancy", and it is not surprising that the bitch may show some of the signs associated with pregnancy, most commonly mammary enlargement and nest making. The extent to which these signs are manifest clinically varies markedly between individuals. Cats can also become pseudopregnant, following a non-fertile mating. (Unlike dogs, of course, cats do not have corpora lutea unless they mate.) The corpus luteum has a limited life hence pseudopregnancy, like true pregnancy, only lasts for a restricted period.

4. **Anoestrus:** Since there is little difference, externally, in the bitch between dioestrus and anoestrus it is difficult to state precisely when one period ends and the next begins, unless one can measure hormone levels in the blood. Anoestrus lasts betwen 4 to 5 months, and during this period there is involution of the uterus. At the same time another wave of ovarian follicles is slowly developing in preparation for commencement of pro-oestrus of the next cycle. Obviously anoestrus normally features only in seasonal breeders; non-seasonal breeders re-cycle from dioestrus to pro-oestrus.

Bitches differ considerably in the regularity of oestrus, but it usually occurs every 6 to 8 months. There are always exceptions to any rules, and an inter-oestrus interval of 12 months is not uncommon.

The first oestrous cycle normally starts soon after puberty which usually occurs at between 6 and 11 months of age. However, there are marked variations between breeds, and some bitches do not commence cycling until they are 2 years old.

(Note that few words cause more confusion of spelling than oestrus: oestrus is a period of heat but as an adjective it is oestrous as in oestrous cycle. In America oestrus/oestrous become estrus/estrous (just as haemoglobin becomes hemoglobin, etc.)

THE QUEEN

In the queen there are multiple periods of oestrus during the breeding season, provided she does not become pregnant. In the non-mated cat the oestrous cycle comprises:

1. **Pro-oestrus:** There are few external signs noticeable during this period of ovarian follicular growth and development. Unlike the bitch there is neither a vaginal discharge nor vulval swelling. During pro-oestrus the queen may be more attractive to the tomcat, but will not allow copulation.

2. **Oestrus:** The period of sexual receptivity, during which the queen is restless, tends to rub her body constantly and "calls" by vocalising, often very loudly. She adopts a crouching position, arching her bark and deflecting the tail to one side. This can be induced by firm stroking along her spine with one's hand.

191

As described earlier, the queen is an "induced ovulator" and ovulation occurs about 24 to 36 hours after copulation though it may take several matings to induce it. The queen remains receptive following ovulation, and oestrus lasts about 7 days. If she is not mated then oestrus lasts up to 10 days although some Burmese and Siamese cats can have a very prolonged oestrus.

3. **Anoestrus:** The period of sexual rest which follows oestrus if ovulation has not occurred. It lasts anywhere between 3 and 15 days, and is characterised by a return to normal behaviour.

Dioestrus is the period of progesterone domination of the genital tract associated with functioning corpora lutea in the ovary. This only occurs in cats if ovulation has been induced (usually by a tomcat, but it can be produced by mechanical stimulation of the vagina, e.g. using a thermometer). Usually the period of dioestrus corresponds with pregnancy, but in some cases where pregnancy does not occur, e.g. if the tomcat is infertile, there may be development of a state of pseudopregnancy.

The interval between oestrus periods in the queen during the breeding season is 15 to 21 days. The breeding season extends from early spring to September and is governed by day length. It may be extended by the use of artificial light regimes.

Puberty is reached at 6 to 10 months of age, but there are marked variations between breeds of cat.

MATING

Mating, or copulation, will normally only occur during oestrus when the female is receptive to the male. In the dog, there is often courtship behaviour involving the dog and bitch licking each other before the dog mounts the bitch. The penis becomes erect and the glans penis protrudes from the preputial orifice. The penis is introduced into the vagina by a thrusting action. This is soon followed by ejaculation; the fluid which is released is called semen and contains sperm and secretions from the prostate gland. It is deposited in the cranial vagina.

Once the dog has ejaculated he usually dismounts and stands pointing away from the bitch. The penis remains erect and is held in the vagina by contraction of muscles in the vestibular wall. This situation is called tying, and prevents the dog and bitch being separated until blood has been drained from the erectile tissue of the penis, allowing it to become smaller. No attempt should be made to try to separate the animals during this period. Although not causing distress to the animals, it often leads to distress amongst owners who are unaware that it is a perfectly normal occurrence!

During oestrus the queen allows the tomcat to mount her. He usually grasps the skin of her neck with his teeth, to ensure he holds onto her. The erect penis protrudes from the prepuce, revealing the barbs on the glans penis. As it enlarges, the penis comes to face cranioventrally so it is easily introduced into the vagina. During mating the queen often cries loudly. Following

192

ejaculation the tomcat dismounts and the queen lies on her side licking and rubbing herself. During this period (up to 10 minutes) she will be very aggressive to the male if he tries to approach her.

PREGNANCY

The inherent motility of sperm allows them to move up through the cervix and uterus into the uterine tube where fertilisation takes place, leading to the formation of the zygote. Essentially fertilisation serves two functions; firstly, it allows mixing of genetic material from both gametes to produce a new unique genetic constitution with some characteristics similar to each parent. Secondly it triggers the repetitive process of cell division which forms the embryo. If the zygote produces more than one embryo there will be identical twins (or quadruplets or whatever). Normally each zygote produces one embryo (hence in humans non-identical twins result from the simultaneous fertilisation of two ova and thus from two separate zygotes). The zygote passes down into the uterus where it starts to develop by division, producing a small cluster of cells. This becomes 'implanted' onto the lining of the uterus after some delay. Initially, nutrients are supplied by the secretions produced by the uterine glands. With further growth the zygote becomes the embryo; once the simple outline of the animal becomes clear the embryo is called a foetus. Embryology is the study of development of the embryo, a truly fascinating area of developmental biology, but it is covered well in other texts, and will not be considered in detail here.

Nutrition of the embryo is provided by the placenta which forms from special membranes, called the allantochorion, which are an outpouching from the body of the embryo. These membranes lie in close contact with the uterine wall and form the placenta. At the placenta blood from the maternal and embryonic circulations come into close contact (but DO NOT mix) allowing diffusion of oxygen and nutrients from the mother, with passage of carbon dioxide and other waste products of metabolism from the embryo to the mother. Blood vessels run from the placenta in the umbilical cord, entering the embryo at the umbilicus. The placenta also functions as an endocrine gland during pregnancy, producing progesterone and relaxin. In cows and ewes, really close contact between the placenta and the uterine wall is limited to multiple button-like attachments.

In both dogs and cats the placenta is cylindrical in shape and encircles the embryo; this arrangement is termed zonary placentation. At the edges of the placenta there is an area called the marginal haematoma. It contains haem pigments derived from degraded maternal red blood cells. This area is green in the bitch and brown in the queen, and is responsible for the coloured discharge observed at parturition when the placenta separates. The reason that the maternal and embryonic blood cannot be allowed to mix directly is that the embryo and the dam are genetically distinct and the white cells of each would attack the other as an 'invader'.

With continuing development the embryo begins to resemble the adult form. In these later stages of development the embryo is called the foetus, and the surrounding membranes are called the foetal membranes. They enclose the foetus in a fluid-filled sac, providing additional mechanical protection. At the time of parturition, when the foetal membranes rupture, these fluids are an important source of lubrication for the expulsion of the foetus.

Both the bitch and queen release many ova at the time of ovulation and there is usually development of several embryos in one pregnancy. Some may die early in the pregnancy, and are usually resorbed by the mother. If all the embryos die pregnancy will end and the uterine contents are aborted through the open cervix.

The duration of pregnancy varies. Traditionally, pregnancy in the bitch and queen was stated to last 63 days. However, it is not unusual for pregnancy to last 70 days without causing any undue problems.

Detection of Pregnancy

The detection and diagnosis of pregnancy can often be difficult, since many of the behavioural changes associated with pregnancy also occur during normal dioestrus. The methods available for detection of pregnancy in the bitch are:

1. **Abdominal palpation,** to feel the enlarging uterus. This may be performed from 3 weeks after mating, when the enlarged uterus may be felt as a "string of pears". However, the ease of uterine palpation varies between animals.

2. **Radiography:** the mineralising foetal skeleton may be seen on abdominal radiographs from day 45 of pregnancy.

3. **Ultrasonography:** this technique is finding increasing application to veterinary medicine, and allows detection of pregnancy from as early as day 18 after mating. Ultrasonography is safer, both for animal and operator, compared with radiography.

MAMMARY DEVELOPMENT

The mammary glands (Chapter 2) enlarge during pregnancy and start to produce milk a few days before parturition. Their development is controlled by a number of hormones, including oestrogen, progesterone and prolactin (Chapter 9).

PARTURITION AND BEYOND

Parturition, or birth, is the co-ordinated expulsion of the foetus, and foetal membranes, from the uterus. It involves both hormonal and neural control mechanisms. Relaxin, a hormone produced by the placenta, causes relaxation and opening of the cervix and also primes the myometrium to respond to oxytocin released by the posterior pituitary gland during parturition.

Parturition is associated with certain behavioural changes. The bitch seeks isolation, becoming restless and panting. She will try to make a nest where she can give birth comfortably. During parturition, separation of the placenta leads to a green vaginal discharge. This is followed by forceful contractions of both the myometrium and the muscles of the abdominal wall. The foetus is expelled from the uterus, through the cervix, vagina and vestibule, and out through the vulva. The placenta is expelled later, and is usually eaten by the bitch.

194

The 'first stage' of labour is the preparation to expel the (first) foetus, involving increased activity of uterine muscle (but no visible straining), relaxation of the cervix and restlessness (discomfort). The foetus also becomes active, moving from the foetal position (compact) to the extended position necessary for birth.

'Second stage' labour is expulsion of the foetus with visible straining (abdominal contraction) reinforcing the uterine activity. 'Third stage' is the expulsion of the placenta ('afterbirth'). Obviously these terms are derived from humans where there is usually a single birth; with multiple births the separation of stages, especially second and third, is rather more artificial. In fact the birth of one puppy or kitten helps the next because as it passes through the birth canal it reflexly stimulates the release of oxytocin from the posterior pituitary. This reinforces uterine contraction and stimulates milk release. Suckling triggers a similar reflex, so assisting the birth of the later members of the litter.

We tend to think of parturition as a relatively violent transition from a totally secure environment to one which, despite maternal protection, is much less secure. But the foetus does not suddenly begin its functions at birth. Its heart will have been beating ever since it first formed and will have circulated the foetal blood (which has haemoglobin with a greater affinity for oxygen since the maternal blood reaching the placenta does not maintain such an oxygen-rich supply as the lungs eventually will). The lungs, of course, are collapsed otherwise they would be filled with fluid and they remain so until the all-important first breath is taken after birth. Often this is helped by the stimulation of the mother's licking (or, in emergencies, by humans slapping the newborn, or blowing into its nostrils, etc). Until birth the lungs are mainly by-passed by most of the cardiac output thanks to special foetal vessels such as the ductus arteriosus. They close soon after birth (but until they do, they may produce audible abnormal murmurs during auscultation with a stethoscope). Licking not only helps to simulate the first breath, it also dries the newborn and encourages the formation of the behavioural bond between dam and offspring. Often the first step is to sever the umbilical cord as the newborn may be still attached to its 'unborn' placenta.

The foetus has already started to exercise its limb muscles well ahead of birth and will also have started to swallow some of the amniotic fluid in which it lies. As a result, its kidneys will have begun to function, though only partially, but enough to produce some urine – which re-enters the amniotic fluid. Even the taste buds are active before birth. None of this should surprise us for unlike babies or puppies or kittens which are extremely helpless (even blind) at birth, many newborn animals, especially herbivores, have to be ready for action almost as soon as they emerge.

Nevertheless, the newborn is crucially dependent on the dam for its nutrition and especially for the protective antibodies contained in the first milk (or colostrum). These are only absorbed by the intestine efficiently in the first few hours after birth though subsequently they may still provide local protection for the intestine. Some of these antibodies may interfere with vaccination, hence the delay before the first injection. Milk, of course, also provides an ideal food for the rapidly growing offspring; at this stage its nutritional demands are maximal not only for growth but temperature regulation, yet it is too weak and currently too inexperienced to obtain its own food. This bond between the mother and offspring also guarantees that close contact is maintained for an extended period which allows for learning behaviour and – with multiple offspring – for play, learning, and social behaviour between littermates. Naturally the mother continues to provide warmth and protection to varying extents and for varying periods, according to species. But in all species this neonatal period is not only a matter of providing a secure physical environment, it is also a vital period of behavioural development with lasting influence on matters such as socialisation, future maternal behaviour, etc.

We all too easily forget that even in animals the maternal role goes far beyond milk, warmth and protection. Indeed, although we often think of parturition as the end point of reproduction it is merely the end of pregnancy. The process of reproduction, which begins with ovulation, is not complete until weaning – the production of a physiologically self-sufficient individual. Even then, especially in social animals, the individual is not yet behaviourally mature and the outstanding example, of course, occurs in humans where some aspects of parental care often extend over as long as 20 years – frequently to the annoyance of the 'offspring'!

The term 'dystocia' refers to difficulty of parturition, and can be due to a variety of factors which may be maternal or foetal. An example of a maternal factor would be a fractured pelvis in the bitch which had healed, causing a narrowing of the pelvic canal. By contrast, an example of a foetal factor is a very large foetus which is too big to pass through the cervix (as with some of the more recent cross-bred types of calves, with the emphasis on an abnormally increased muscle mass). Obviously foetal factors are more likely to precipitate dystocia in species with fewer (larger) offspring.

Pregnancy is maintained by hormones from the pituitary (notably prolactin) and corpus luteum (progesterone); the placenta also produces progesterone. This hormone suppresses the oestrous cycle during pregnancy and similar drugs are used to suppress it artificially. The cat is unusual in that it can come into oestrus even during pregnancy. Most species come back into oestrus soon after parturition, i.e. early in lactation (unlike the human menstrual cycle which is often suppressed throughout lactation). In seasonal breeders, however, the next oestrus is usually delayed until the next due breeding season so bitches, cats and ewes, for example, are unlikely to return to oestrus during lactation, though cats often do so a week or two after the litter is weaned. In contrast, dairy cows (which are non-seasonal) are usually pregnant relatively early in lactation, thus reducing the interval between consecutive lactations. Were it not so, the economics of traditional dairy farming would collapse under the weight of cows failing to earn their keep. Exceptionally, cats will mate during lactation, in which case they can be pregnant for most of the year. Clearly nutrition is a vital factor in lactation (and pregnancy), not only to keep pace with the demands of milk production but also to make good any depletion of stores during the previous pregnancy, in preparation for the next.

INDEX

197

Biceps femoris	176
Bile	97, 99, 108-110, 112
Bile duct	96, 99
Binocular vision	145
Bio-assay	125
Birth	54, 181, 194
Bladder	74, 81-85, 131-132, 143
Bleeding	43
Blood	20, 25, 30-32, 34, 39-48, 111
Blood-brain barrier	134
Blood cells	46-48, 157
Blood flow	15, 23-24, 36-37, 39, 45, 57, 61-69, 124, 126
Blood pressure	11, 37, 63-66, 69, 73, 124, 134, 143
Blood supply	62, 100
Blood transfusion	61, 113
Blood types	47, 113
Blood vessels	16-17, 49-50, 61-66, 143
Blood volume	68-69
Bone(s)	7, 31, 57, 121-122, 155, 162
Bone cortex	156-157
Bone damage	72, 80
Bone growth	157
Bone marrow	157
Bone repair	157
Borborygmi	95
Bowman's capsule	73
Brachial artery	55-56
Bradycardia	53
Brain	34, 56, 71, 109, 113, 116-117, 119, 130, 136
Brain blood flow	25, 62-64
Breathing	21, 24-27, 30-32, 35, 67, 134, 172
Breathing difficulties	32
Broad ligament	187-188
Bronchus (i)	26, 29-30, 143
Bronchiole	26, 29-30
Brown fat	36
Buffers	79-80
Bulbourethral glands	85-86
Bursa	172

C	
C cells	121
Caecum	97-98
Calcaneus	170-171
Calcitonin	121-122
Calcium	13, 43-45, 72, 74, 77, 111, 121-122, 155-156, 178
Callus	16, 157
Cancellous bone	156-157
Canine	89
Canthus	145-146
Capillaries	24, 30, 39, 41-42, 45, 49, 58, 61-63, 68-69, 134
Capillary damage	69, 108, 110
Capillary hydrostatic pressure	61, 69
Carbohydrate	24, 36, 106, 109, 112
Carbon dioxide	21-26, 30, 56, 63, 79, 193
Carbonic anhydrose	24
Cardia	93-94
Cardiac muscle	50-69, 171, 179
Cardiac output	61, 64-66, 72
Cardiac rhythm	67-68
Cardiac sphincter	93, 109
Cardiovascular system	49-69
Caries	89
Carnassial teeth	89

207

Secretin	110
Secretion	75, 106-107, 109-110, 114, 125
Semen	84, 183, 192
Semicircular canals	151-152
Seminiferous tubules	119, 124, 183
Semimembranosus muscle	176
Semitendinosus muscle	176
Sensory receptors	16-17, 130
Sensory nerves (afferent)	127, 131
Septum	53-54
Serum	44-45
Sesamoid bone	158, 171, 174-175
Set point	10-11, 33-34, 37
Sex hormones	119, 123-124
Sexual receptiveness	181, 190-191
Shiver	36-37, 172
Shock	34, 37, 68-69, 79, 108, 110
Short bone	158
Shoulder joint	167-168
Silent heat	190
Sinoatrial node (SA)	67, 179
Sinus	27-28, 89
Sinus arrhythmia	67
Sinus rhythm	67, 179
Skeletal muscle	32, 57, 127, 132, 145, 171, 176, 179
Skeleton	155, 162
Skin	13-20, 34, 36-37, 57, 104, 122
Skin glands	13-15
Skull	132, 159, 162
Sleep	136
Small intestine	95-98, 109
Smell	27, 135, 138, 145, 153
Smooth muscle	19, 57, 82, 94-95, 98, 109, 127, 132, 143, 148, 171, 179, 188
Sneezing	27
Sniffing	153
Sodium	39-41, 64, 72-73, 76-81, 104, 107-108, 111, 121, 123-124, 126, 128
Sodium-potassium pump	39-41
Soft palate	27-28, 30, 87, 92
Solubility	86
Solutes	40-41
Somatic nervous system	127, 132
Somatotropin	117
Sound	29, 150, 152
Special senses	132, 135, 145-153
Specific gravity	76
Sperm	84, 119, 124, 181, 183, 193
Spermatic cord	182-184
Spermatogenesis	183
Speying	103
Sphincters	62, 68, 93, 97, 109
Spinal cord	130-136, 164
Spinal injury	81, 99, 137
Spinal nerve	132, 136, 139-141
Spinal reflex	81
Spinous process	164-165
Spleen	60-61
Spontaneous ovulation	186
Stasis	110
Steatorrhoea	109
Sternbrae	31
Sternum	101, 166
Steroids	126
Stifle joint	160, 170-171